DYSPEPSIA - ADVANCES IN UNDERSTANDING AND MANAGEMENT

Edited by **Eldon Shaffer** and **Michael Curley**

Dyspepsia - Advances in Understanding and Management
http://dx.doi.org/10.5772/50862
Edited by Eldon Shaffer and Michael Curley

Contributors

Sylvester Chuks Nwokediuko, Ratha-Korn Vilaichone, Durre Sabih, Kashif Rahim, Jan Pen, Mónica Roxo-Rosa, Mónica Oleastro, Ana Isabel Lopes, Wojciech Leppert, Yves Muscat Baron, Winnie Nelson, Craig Coleman, Christine Kohn, Jeffrey Kluger, Joyce LaMori, Jeffrey Schein, Schurman, Craig Friesen, Eldon Shaffer

Published by InTech

Janeza Trdine 9, 51000 Rijeka, Croatia

Publishing Process Manager Danijela Duric
Technical Editor InTech DTP team
Cover InTech Design team

Additional hard copies can be obtained from orders@intechopen.com

Dyspepsia - Advances in Understanding and Management, Edited by Eldon Shaffer and Michael Curley
p. cm.
ISBN 978-953-51-1205-1

For EU product safety concerns:
IN TECH d.o.o., Prolaz Marije Krucifikse Kozulić 3, 51000 Rijeka, Croatia,
info@intechopen.com or visit our website at intechopen.com.

Meet the editors

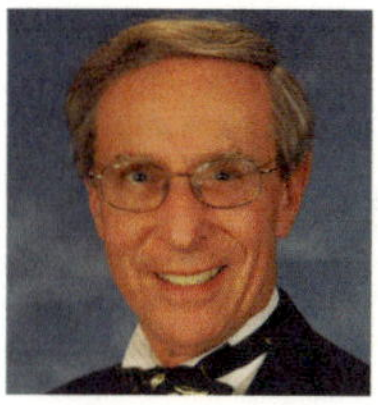

Eldon Shaffer is a Gastroenterologist who has held leadership positions in academic Medicine. At a university level, Dr. Shaffer was founding Division Head (Gastroenterology); founding chair, Gastrointestinal Research Group; Associate Dean (Clinical Affairs) and Department Head (Internal Medicine), all in the Faculty of Medicine, University of Calgary. At a national level, he was the founding President of the Canadian Association for Study of the Liver (CASL); President, Canadian Association of Gastroenterology (CAG); President, Canadian Society for Clinical Investigation (CSCI); Chair of the Medical Advisory Board, Crohn's and Colitis Foundation and President, Canadian Professors of Medicine. At an international level, he served on committees for the American College of Gastroenterology; the American Association for the Study of Liver Disease; the American Gastroenterological Association, chairing its Liver Biliary section and sitting on the AGA Council, and the Organizing Committee (Chair, Public Relations Committee) for the World Congress of Gastroenterology (Montreal 2005). His personal research activity has yielded over 500 papers, abstracts and edited texts. A recognized educator, Dr. Shaffer has received awards nationally from the CAG, CASL, CSCI. He currently is a Professor of Medicine in the Division of Gastroenterology and Hepatology, University of Calgary, where he enjoys an active consulting practice in Gastroenterology and continues to maintain his education and research interests that span from hepatobiliary diseases though functional gut disease and eosinophilic gastrointestinal disease.

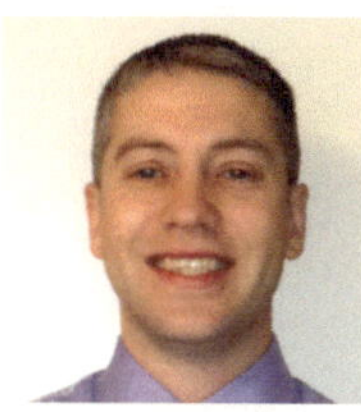

Michael Curley grew up in Cornwall, Prince Edward Island, Canada. He did his medical training including residencies in Internal Medicine and Gastroenterology at Dalhousie University, Halifax, Nova Scotia. He is a consultant Gastroenterologist and clinical assistant professor with the Division of Gastroenterology and Hepatology at the University of Calgary, South Health Campus, Calgary, Alberta. His main clinical interests include upper gastrointestinal tract motility disorders and functional disorders. He has a strong interest in medical education and has an active role in mentoring and teaching trainees from medical student to Gastroenterology fellowship level.

Contents

Preface

Dyspepsia suggests impaired digestion but when chronic, implies recurrent upper abdominal pain or fullness that may follow a meal. Functional dyspepsia lacks evidence of a structural basis, yet is a common disorder that often profoundly impacts the patient's quality of life. Many clinicians have a relatively poor understanding of factors that play a role in this disorder. Differentiation between organic disease and functional dyspepsia is often difficult. Further confounding this is their occasional co-existence. Management of patients with functional dyspepsia can be frustrating, particularly as symptoms are frequently refractory.

This textbook is specifically written for clinicians involved in managing patients with dyspepsia. It is a practical guide with up-to-date suggestions on evaluation, diagnosis, and management from experts from around the world. Each chapter is a succinct review of current topics that play a role in the pathogenesis and management of this disorder. Special populations such as pediatrics, those with cardiovascular disease and women's health are specifically examined.

Dyspepsia: Advances in Understanding and Management is essential reading for those who wish to advance their understanding of this complex and often challenging disorder.

We dedicate this book to our significant others, our families and those suffering from functional dyspepsia.

Eldon Shaffer
Professor of Medicine
Division of Gastroenterology and Hepatology, University of Calgary
Canada

Michael Curley
Consultant Gastroenterologist and clinical assistant professor
Division of Gastroenterology and Hepatology
University of Calgary
Canada

Chapter 1

Diagnostic Testing for Functional Dyspepsia

Durre Sabih and Muhammad Kashif Rahim

Additional information is available at the end of the chapter

http://dx.doi.org/10.5772/57088

1. Introduction

Dyspepsia is defined as predominantly midline pain or discomfort located in the upper abdomen [1]. Discomfort refers to a subjective, negative feeling that is not "painful". Dyspepsia can incorporate a variety of symptoms including early satiety or upper abdominal fullness. Although the term implies a relationship with eating and the majority of patients have symptoms worsened by food, this is no longer necessary to diagnose dyspepsia [2]. During the investigation of dyspepsia, three major structural causes are readily identifiable: peptic ulcer disease (10%), gastroesophageal reflux (20%) (with or without esophagitis), and malignancy (2%) [3]. Thus, most (50%-70%) patients with chronic dyspepsia do not have a significant focal or structural lesion found at endoscopy. When symptoms are chronic or recurrent (table 1) but without an identifiable structural cause using standard diagnostic tests (usually endoscopy), the condition is usually labelled functional or functional dyspepsia [4, 5]. Hence functional dyspepsia is a diagnosis of exclusion, the implication being that symptoms have been investigated without demonstrating an organic or anatomical cause [5].

Functional dyspepsia is not life-threatening and is not associated with any increase in mortality. However, the impact of this condition on patients and health care services is considerable. In a recent community survey of several European and North American populations, 20% of people with dyspeptic symptoms had consulted either primary care physicians or hospital specialists; more than 50% of dyspepsia sufferers were on medication most of the time and approximately 30% reported taking days off from work or school due to their symptoms [5, 6]. Patients with functional dyspepsia have a significantly reduced quality of life when compared to the general population [7].

The Rome III criteria for diagnosing functional dyspepsia are persistent or recurrent upper abdominal pain or discomfort for a period of 12 weeks, which need not be consecutive, in the preceding 12 months, with symptoms present more than 25 percent of the time, and an absence

Symptom	Definition	
Pain centered in the upper abdomen	Pain refers to a subjective, unpleasant sensation; some patients may feel that tissue damage is occurring. Other pain sensations could be throbbing, shooting, stabbing, cramping, gnawing, burning or aching. By questioning the patient, pain should be distinguished from discomfort.	
Discomfort centered in the upper abdomen	A subjective, unpleasant sensation or feeling that is not interpreted as pain according to the patient and which, if fully assessed, can include any of the symptoms below.	
	Early satiety	A feeling that the stomach is overfilled soon after starting to eat, out of proportion to the size of the meal being eaten, so that the meal cannot be finished.
	Fullness after meal	Unpleasant sensations like the persistence of food in the stomach; this may or may not occur post-prandially (slow digestion).
	Bloating in the upper abdomen	Tightness located in the upper abdomen; it should be distinguished from visible abdominal distension.
	Nausea	Queasiness or sick sensation; a feeling of the need to vomit.

Table 1. The spectrum of dyspepsia symptoms and recommended definitions [4, 5]

of clinical, biochemical, endoscopic, and ultrasonographic evidence of organic disease that would account for the symptoms [1] (Table 2).

12 weeks minimum, that need not be consecutive, in the preceding 12 months of:
• Persistent or recurrent symptoms (pain or discomfort centred in the upper abdomen);
• No evidence of organic disease (including at upper GI endoscopy) that is likely to explain the symptoms;
• No evidence that dyspepsia is exclusively relieved by defecation or associated with the onset of a change in stool frequency or stool form (i.e., not irritable bowel).

Table 2. Rome III diagnostic criteria for functional dyspepsia [1, 9]

On the basis of the most bothersome or predominant single symptom, identified by the patient, functional dyspepsia is further classified into various subgroups [4, 9]:

1. Ulcer-like dyspepsia

Pain centred in the upper abdomen is the predominant (most bothersome) symptom [9].

2. Dysmotility-like dyspepsia

An unpleasant or troublesome non-painful sensation (discomfort) centred in the upper abdomen is the predominant symptom; this sensation may be characterized by or associated with upper abdominal fullness, early satiety, bloating, or nausea [9].

3. Unspecified (non-specific) dyspepsia

Symptoms do not fulfil the criteria for ulcer-like or dysmotility-like dyspepsia [9].

http://dx.doi.org/10.5772/57088

2. Functional dyspepsia: Pathophysiologic mechanisms and their relation to symptom pattern

Several pathophysiologic mechanisms explain underlie dyspeptic symptoms. These include delayed gastric emptying, impaired gastric accommodation to a meal, and hypersensitivity to gastric distension, *H. pylori* infection, altered response to duodenal lipids or acid, abnormal duodenojejunal motility, or central nervous system dysfunction. At present, the pathophysiology of functional dyspepsia is only partially elucidated. However, there is growing evidence that functional dyspepsia is in fact a very heterogeneous disorder and different subgroups can be identified based on different demographic, clinical, and pathophysiologic features [2].

1. Delayed gastric emptying

Delayed gastric emptying is traditionally considered a major pathophysiologic mechanism underlying symptoms in functional dyspepsia and idiopathic gastroparesis [10]. Several large single-centre studies from Europe found association between delayed gastric emptying and the prevalence and severity of symptoms like post-prandial fullness, nausea, and vomiting [10]. Similarly, other reports have investigated the relationship between delayed gastric emptying and symptom pattern and severity [2]. Depending on the study, the percentage of dyspeptic patients with delayed gastric emptying ranges from 20% to 50%. In a meta-analysis of 17 studies involving 868 dyspeptic patients and 397 controls, significant delay of solid gastric emptying was present in almost 40% of patients with functional dyspepsia [11]. Various causes of delayed gastric emptying are summarized in table 3.

2. Impaired gastric accommodation to a meal

The motor functions of the proximal and distal stomach differ remarkably. The proximal stomach (body) serves mainly as a reservoir. In contrast, the distal stomach (antrum) regulates gastric emptying of solids by grinding and sieving the contents until the particles are small enough to pass the pylorus. The stomach accommodates to a meal by relaxing of the proximal stomach, providing the meal with a reservoir and enabling an increase in volume without an increase in pressure. Scintigraphic and ultrasonographic studies have shown an abnormal intragastric distribution of food in patients with functional dyspepsia, with preferential accumulation in the distal stomach. These findings suggest defective postprandial accommodation of the proximal stomach [12, 13].

3. Hypersensitivity to gastric distension

Physiologic stimuli during the digestive process are not normally perceived but in some circumstances may induce conscious sensations. Patients with functional gastrointestinal diseases may have a sensory dysfunction of the gut (termed visceral hypersensitivity), with normal physiological stimuli perceived as discomfort or pain [14]. Patients with functional dyspepsia appear to have enhanced sensitivity to gastric distension [10, 15, 16].

4. Altered duodenal sensitivity to lipids or acid

The symptoms of dyspepsia are usually exacerbated by meals which are rich in fat [20]. Similarly the duodenum is more sensitive to acid in those with functional dyspepsia. The duodenal motor response to acid is decreased in patients with functional dyspepsia, resulting in reduced clearance of exogenous duodenal acid [21].

5. Inflammation

About a third of patients with irritable bowel syndrome or dyspepsia describe the onset of symptoms after an acute enteric infection. It is possible that mucosal inflammation may have a part in the creation of the visceral hypersensitivity.

6. H. Pylori infection

The discovery of *H. pylori* led to uncovering a causal relationship between *H. pylori* infection and the occurrence of duodenal and gastric ulcers [17]. The role of *H. pylori* is less clear in functional dyspepsia. Systematic reviews of the epidemiologic evidence on a relationship between *H. pylori* infection and functional dyspepsia have found no evidence for a strong association [18, 19].

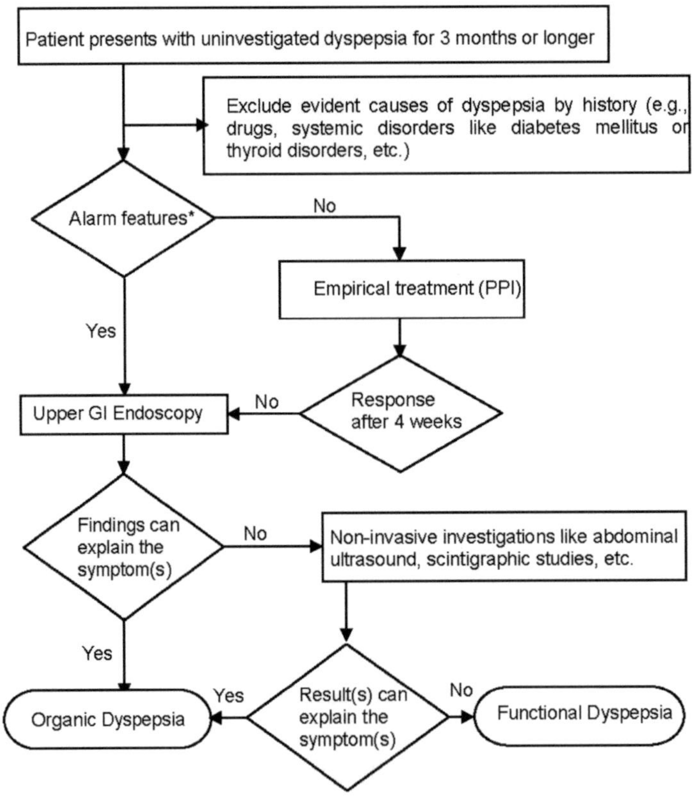

*The alarm features are unintended weight loss, progressive dysphagia, recurrent or persistent vomiting, evidence of gastrointestinal bleeding, anemia, fever, family history of gastric cancer, new onset dyspepsia in the subjects over 40 years of age in population with high prevalence of upper gastrointestinal malignancy and over 45 and 50 years in populations with intermediate and low prevalence, respectively. **Adapted from reference [22]

Figure 1. Diagnostic algorithm for functional (functional) dyspepsia**

3. Causes of delayed gastric emptying

The various causes that are related to delayed gastric emptying are summarized here in Table 3 [23].

Acute (Transient) Delayed Gastric Emptying	Cigarette smoking, Alcohol, Viral gastroenteritis, Hyperglycemia, Acidosis, Hypokalemia, Immobilization, Myxoedema, Hypocalcaemia, Hypercalaemia, Hypomagnesaemia, Hepatic coma, Postoperative ileus, Parenteral nutrition,
Chronic Delayed Gastric Emptying	Gastric ulcer disease, Functional dyspepsia, Gastroesophageal reflux disease, Diabetes Mellitus, Hypothyroidism, Post gastric surgery, Addison's diseases, Pernicious anaemia, Achlorhydria, Connective tissue diseases, Anorexia nervosa, Depression, Neurologic disorders (Multiple sclerosis, Parkinsonism, paraneoplastic syndrome etc).
Pharmacological Agents and Hormones	Antacids (aluminium hydroxide), Opiates, Anticholinergics, Tricyclic antidepressants, Beta adrenergic agonists, Levodopa, Calcium channel blockers, Progesterone, Birth control pills, Gastrin, Cholecystokinin, Somatostatin

Table 3. Causes of Delayed Gastric Emptying [23].

4. Diagnostic investigations of dyspepsia

Functional dyspepsia is usually a diagnosis of exclusion; the diagnosis is made after eliminating organic disease or a structural basis for symptoms. The physician must decide how many investigations to order before deciding that the patient has a functional disorder (Table 4). The heterogeneity of presentation and the extensive differential diagnosis including significant organic disease mandates rapid exclusion of pathologies like peptic ulcer disease, reflux esophagitis and malignancy of the stomach or esophagus. Another perspective is the test-and-treat approach that includes acid suppression, treatment of *H.pylori* infection and early endoscopy. Patients with "alarm features" (Fig 1), or those older than 40-50 years (depending on ethnicity) require a more aggressive strategy such as early endoscopy. It must also be understood that there are many patients who can have both organic as well as functional components of dyspepsia.

Initial investigations may include blood counts, electrolytes, fasting blood sugar, renal function tests and thyroid function tests. Testing for celiac disease and stool examination for occult blood or parasites may also be considered. *H.pylori* infection can be diagnosed by serology, breath or stool testing.

Gastric accommodation can be assessed by gastric barotest. The barotest measures gastric tone and comprises of a bag that can be maintained at a constant pressure by feedback mechanisms (termed a barostat). Volume changes in the bag thus represent variation in gut - the bag becomes bigger with gut relaxation and smaller with contraction. "Barotesting" is the "gold standard" for visceral hypersensitivity, but is invasive and uncomfortable, so non-invasive means have been developed that include SPECT (Single Photon Emission Tomography) imaging and 3-D ultrasound.

SPECT can be used to assess intragastric volume although correlation with barotest has not been consistently established and the volumes determined do not reflect muscle activity of the stomach. 3D ultrasound can also be used for volume determination of the stomach but this remains a highly operator dependent technique and there is limited data available in the literature.

Chemical hypersensitivity tests can be done by a duodenal infusion of lipid to provoke early symptoms of gastric distension in patients with functional dyspepsia and relief by administering a cholecystokinin receptor antagonist (loxiglumide). CCK-8 (cholecystokinin octapeptide) intravenously can be used instead of the lipid infusion to provoke symptoms in patients with functional dyspepsia, but this does not affect normal individuals.

Scintigraphic imaging lends itself elegantly to the evaluation of functional-dyspepsia due to the inherent strength of dynamic imaging and generating physiological data. Currently, it remains the only method to quantitatively measure the rate of gastric emptying.

Gastric scintigraphy employs a radiolabeled meal to measure emptying [24]. Gastric scintigraphy has evolved to include an evaluation of compartmental or antral motility, and more recently to SPECT to evaluate postprandial gastric accommodation. As a physiologic, quantitative, and non-invasive test, gastric emptying scintigraphy is well suited for evaluating patients before and after medical or surgical treatment. This procedure is now widely considered the gold standard for evaluating gastric emptying. The advantages of radionuclide imaging are:

1. The method is simple and non-invasive from the patient's point of view, requiring a single oral administration of the radionuclide.
2. The meal used in this method is physiological and does not alter the normal physiology of the gut.
3. Reaction to the radiopharmaceutical is rare.
4. Both solid and liquid meals can be studied and the gastric emptying can be quantified.
5. The radiation dose is very low so that repeated studies can be done to follow the progress of the disease or the response to treatment and the method can therefore be used as a research tool.
6. This method can be used to assess the amount of original meal in the stomach irrespective of the gastric secretions or the duodenal reflux.
7. There is no documented complication reported as the result of the gastric emptying studies.
8. There are different protocols with a 2, 3 or 4 hour end points (3 and 4 hour end points are emerging as more diagnostic).

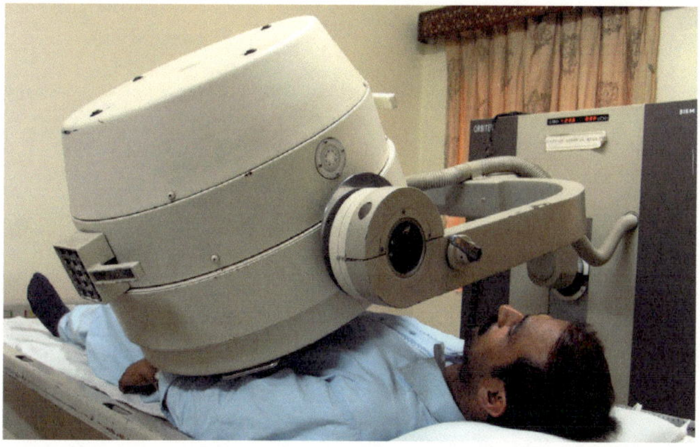

Figure 2. Position of patient and camera during acquisition of images for scintigraphic evaluation of gastric emptying times.

Test	Strengths	Weaknesses
Radiological method (Barium meal)	• Gastroparesis can be diagnosed with barium meal	• Contraindicated in acid peptic disease and partial intestinal obstruction • Can cause barium appendicitis
Ultrasonography	• Non invasive • Does not involve ionizing radiation • Equipment used is available in most of the hospitals	• Operator dependent • Relatively time consuming as it requires repeated and prolonged observations
Endoscopy	• Permits direct visualization of the oesophagus, gastric and duodenal mucosa • First-line diagnostic procedure for patients with alarm features	• Invasive procedure • Not well accepted by patients • Requires trained personnel • Limited availability of equipment
Gastric emptying scintigraphy	• Simple and non-invasive • Physiological meal used • No reaction to pharmaceutical • No documented complication	• Ionizing radiation used • Time consuming • Equipment widely available • Degree of delayed gastric emptying does not correlate well with symptomatology
C-13 Acetate breath test	• Non invasive • No radiation involved • Can be adapted for solid or liquid emptying (C-13 sodium acetate for liquid and C-13 octanoic acid for solids)	• Variability similar to other tests • Good reproducibility • Needs special equipment (mass spectrophotometer) but cheaper alternates have been developed (NDIRS* and LARA**)

*NDIRS Non-dispersive isotope-selective infrared spectroscopy

**LARA Laser-assisted ratio analysis

Table 4. Investigations for the work-up of functional dyspepsia with their strengths and weaknesses

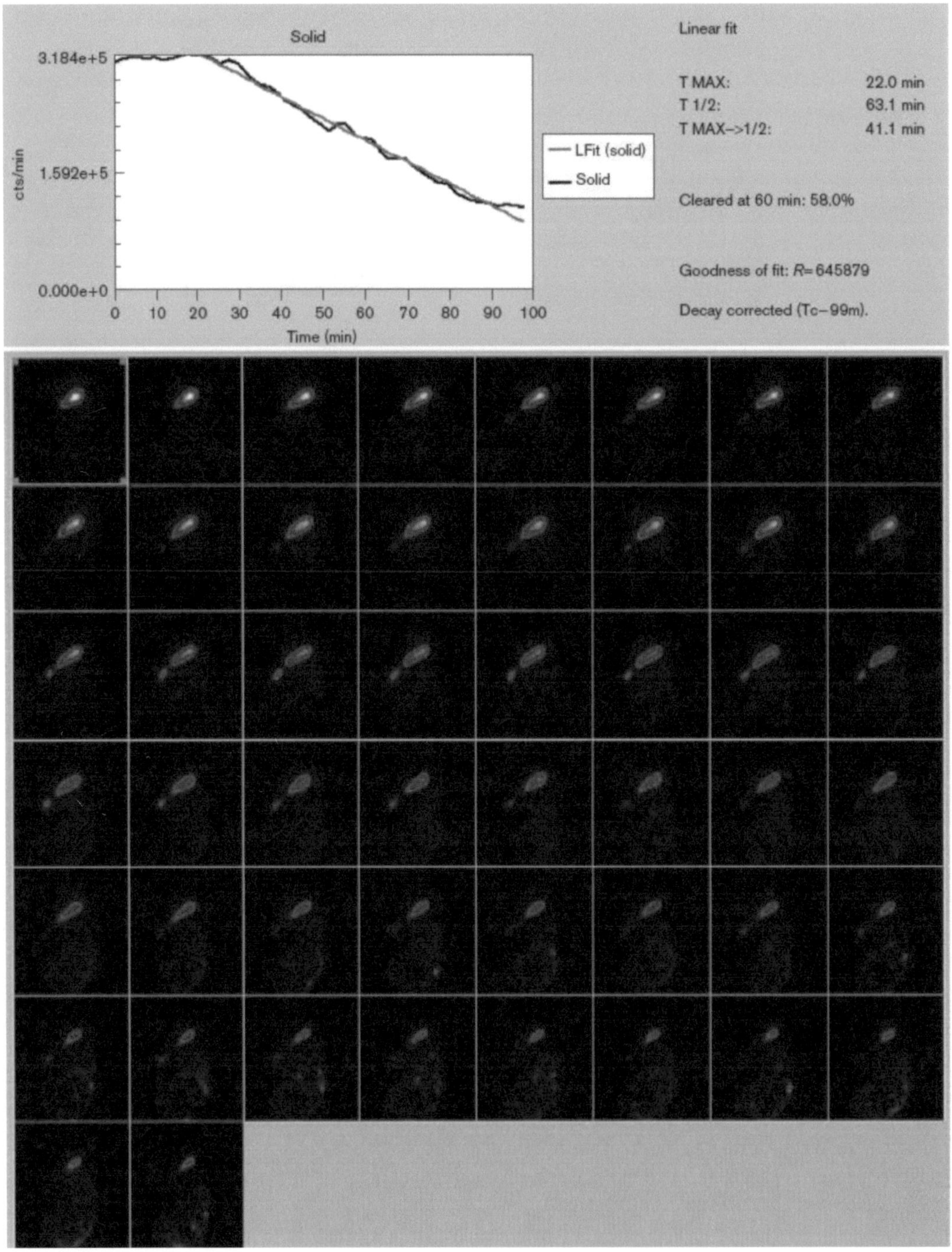

Figure 3. Figure Dynamic images and time–activity curves of a normal person.

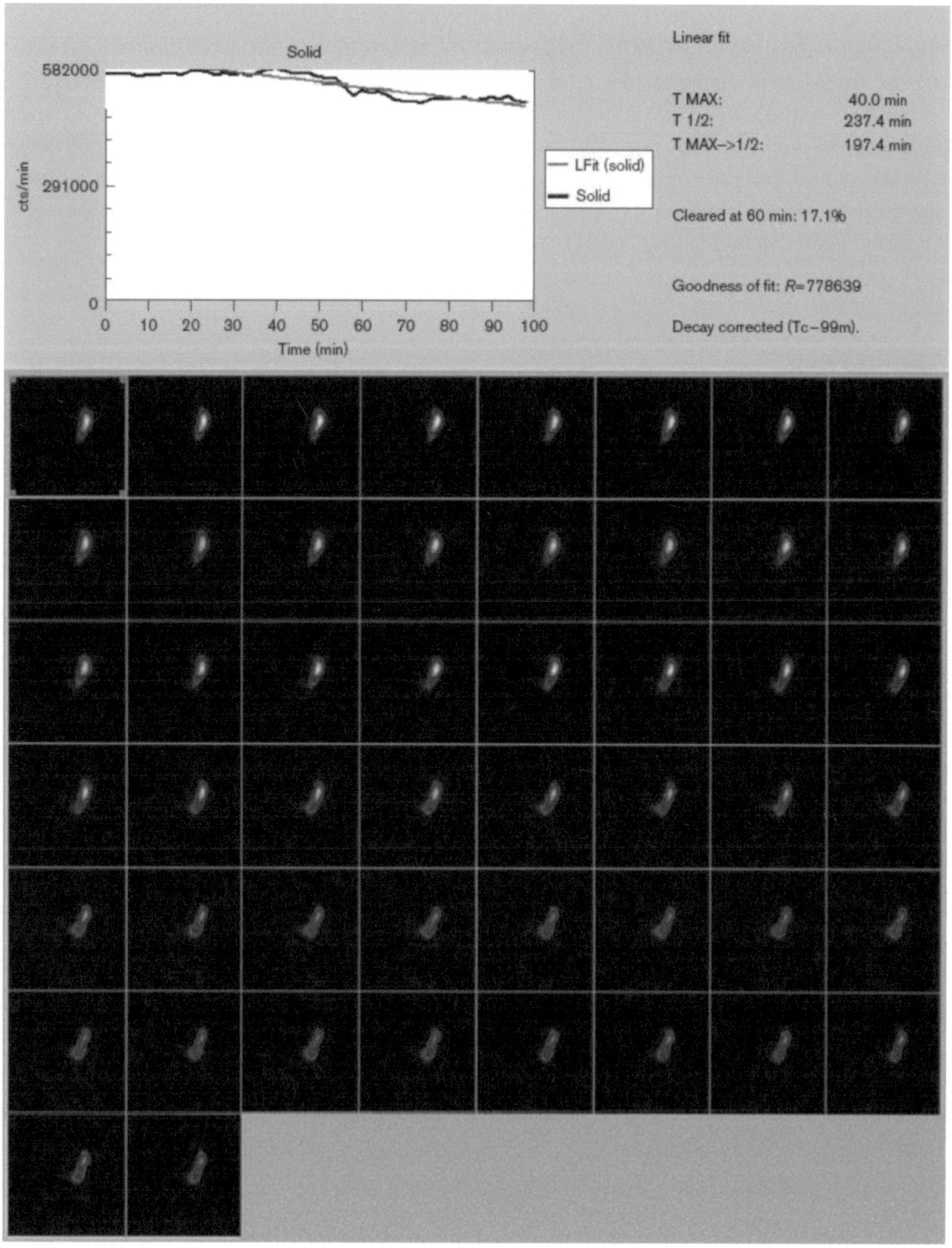

Figure 4. Dynamic images and time–activity curves of a patient with impaired gastric emptying.

5. Conclusion

Functional dyspepsia is a common problem with a significant impact on individuals and society. A variety of diagnostic tests are available to exclude organic disease and characterize underlying pathophysiologic abnormalities. Further work is needed to validate existing diagnostic tests in different populations. The goal of having an objective test that correlates with the symptom severity remains elusive. Physicians must remain cognisant that functional disorders create the same or perhaps even more distress in the patient when compared to conditions that can yield evidence of organic pathology.

Author details

Durre Sabih[1] and Muhammad Kashif Rahim[2]

*Address all correspondence to: dsabih@yahoo.com

1 Multan Institute of Nuclear Medicine and Radiotherapy (MINAR), Nishtar Medical College and Hospital, Multan, Pakistan

2 Multan Institute of Nuclear Medicine and Radiotherapy (MINAR), Nishtar Medical College and Hospital, Multan, Pakistan

References

[1] Talley NJ, Colin-Jones D, Koch KL, Koch M, Nyren O, et al. Functional dyspepsia: a classification with guidelines of diagnosis and management. Gastroenterol Int 1991; 4:145–160.

[2] Tack J, Bisschops R, Sarnelli G. Pathophysiology and treatment of functional dyspepsia. Gastroenterology 2004; 127: 1239-1255

[3] Talley NJ, Vakil NB, Moayyedi P. American gastroenterological association technical review on the evaluation of dyspepsia. Gastroenterology 2005; 129: 1756-1780

[4] Talley NJ, Stanghellini V, Heading RC, Koch KL, Malagelada JR, et al. Functional gastroduodenal disorders. Gut 1999; 45:37–42.

[5] Baker G, Fraser RJ, Young G. Subtypes of functional dyspepsia. World J Gastroenterol 2006; 12(17): 2667-2671

[6] Haycox A, Einarson T, Eggleston A. The health economic impact of upper gastrointestinal symptoms in the general population: results from the Domestic/International

Gastroenterology Surveillance Study (DIGEST). Scand J Gastroenterol 1999; 231 Suppl: 38-47

[7] Moayyedi P, Mason J. Clinical and economic consequences of dyspepsia in the community. Gut 2002; 50 Suppl 4: iv10-iv12

[8] Chang L. Review article: epidemiology and quality of life in functional gastrointestinal disorders. Aliment Pharmacol Ther 2004; 20 Suppl 7: 31-39

[9] Tack J, Nicholas J.T,Camilleri M, Holtmann G, Hu P,Malagelada JR, Stanghellini V et al Functional. Functional Gastroduodenal disorders. Gastroenterology 2006; 130:1466-1469.

[10] nepeel P, Geypens B, Janssens J, Tack J. Symptoms associated with impaired gastric emptying of solids and liquids in functional dyspepsia. Am J Gastroenterol 2003; 98: 783–788.

[11] Waldron B, Cullen PT, Kumar R, et al. Evidence for hypomotility in functional dyspepsia: a prospective multifactorial study. Gut 1991; 32:246–251.

[12] Ricci R, Bontempo I, La Bella A, De Tschudy A, Corazziari E. Dyspeptic symptoms and gastric antrum distribution. An ultrasonographic study. Ital J Gastroenterol 1987; 19:215–217.

[13] Gilja OH, Hausken T, Wilhelmsen I, Berstad A. Impaired accommodation of proximal stomach to a meal in functional dyspepsia. Dig Dis Sci 1996; 41:689–696.

[14] Camilleri M, Coulie B, Tack J. Visceral hypersensitivity: facts, speculations and challenges. Gut 2001; 48:125–131.

[15] Boeckxstaens GE, Hirsch DP, Kuiken SD, Heisterkamp SH, Tytgat GN. The proximal stomach and postprandial symptoms in functional dyspeptics. Am J Gastroenterol 2002; 97:40–48.

[16] Tack J, Bisschops R, Caenepeel P, Vos R, Janssens J. Pathophysiological relevance of fasting versus postprandial sensitivity testing in functional dyspepsia (abstr). Gastroenterol 2002; 122; A34.

[17] Thumshirn M, Camilleri M, Saslow SB, Williams DE, Burton DD, Hanson RB. Gastric accommodation in functional dyspepsia and the roles of Helicobacter pylori infection and vagal function. Gut 1999; 44:55–64.

[18] Rhee PL, Kim YH, Son HJ, et al. Lack of association of Helicobacter pylori infection with gastric hypersensitivity or delayed gastric emptying in functional dyspepsia. Am J Gastroenterol 1999; 94: 316–569.

[19] Sarnelli G, Janssens J, Tack J. Helicobacter pylori is not associated with symptoms and pathophysiological mechanisms of functional dyspepsia. Dig Dis Sci 2003; 48:2229–36.

[20] Houghton LA, Mangnall YF, Dwivedi A, Read N. Increased nutrient sensitivity in a subgroup of patients with nonulcer dyspepsia. Gut 1990; 31:1185 (abstract).

[21] Samsom M, Verhagen MA, van Berge Henegouwen GP, Smout AJPM. Abnormal clearance of exogenous acid and increased acid sensitivity of the proximal duodenum in dyspeptic patients. Gastroenterology 1999; 116:515–520.

[22] Miwa H, Ghoshal UC, Gonlachanvit S, et al. Asian Consensus Report on Functional Dyspepsia. J Neurogastroenterol Motil. 2012; 18: 150-68.

[23] Urbain JLC, Maurer AH. The Stomach. In: Wagner HN Jr, Szabo Z, Buchanan JW, eds. Principles of Nuclear Medicine, 2nd edition. Philadelphia: WB Saunders; 1995: 916–929.

[24] Griffith GH, Owen GM, Kirkman S, et al. Measurement of rate of gastric emptying using chromium-51. Lancet 1966; 1:1244–45.

Chapter 2

Is Functional Dyspepsia Idiopathic?

Sylvester Chuks Nwokediuko

Additional information is available at the end of the chapter

http://dx.doi.org/10.5772/56620

1. Introduction

Dyspepsia is currently defined by Rome III criteria for the diagnosis of functional gastrointestinal disorders (FGIDs), as the presence of one or more of the following symptoms: bothersome postprandial fullness, early satiation, epigastric pain and epigastric burning [1] These are symptoms thought to originate from the gastroduodenal region. Bloating and nausea often coexist with dyspepsia but are considered nonspecific and are thus not included in the Rome III criteria. However, there have been attempts by some researchers to broaden this definition to include more symptoms. The Asian consensus guideline includes bloating, nausea, vomiting and belching in the definition of dyspepsia [2]

Dyspeptic patients who have not undergone any investigations are defined as having uninvestigated dyspepsia. An organic cause is found in only a minority who seek medical care [3, 4]. The remaining group is labeled as having functional dyspepsia (FD). Organic dyspepsia means there is a clear anatomic or pathophysiologic reason for the dyspeptic complaints, such as peptic ulcer or cancer. In contrast, when a diagnosis of functional dyspepsia has been made, it means that a number of investigations were performed including upper gastrointestinal endoscopy, and were found to be normal [5].

The need for more systematic description of FGIDs gave rise to the Rome process, which has evolved from Rome I in 1991 [6], Rome II in 1999 [7], to the most recent, which is Rome III [1]. According to Rome I and Rome II definitions, FD was defined as the presence of pain or discomfort centered in the upper abdomen, in the absence of organic disease that readily explained the symptoms [7]. While the meaning of pain is readily understood, the lack of an accurate definition for discomfort was a major limitation of Rome I. Rome I also included reflux symptoms in FD, and recognized a subgroup called "reflux-like dyspepsia". Rome II tried to correct this by excluding patients with predominant heartburn from the definition of FD. Rome

I and Rome II criteria did not account for meal-related symptoms and this was the fundamental change in Rome III criteria [8, 9].

Rome III criteria made a distinction between meal-induced symptoms and meal-unrelated symptoms, and this forms the basis of newly defined subcategories of FD:

1. Meal-induced dyspeptic symptoms (postprandial distress syndrome, which is characterized by postprandial fullness and early satiation)

2. Epigastric pain syndrome or EPS, characterized by epigastric pain and epigastric burning.

The traditional definition of FD portrays it as an idiopathic condition [10]. However, recent studies suggest that this condition have some pathophysiologic correlates. A diversity of changes in gastrointestinal structure and function has been described in this heterogeneous disorder. In this chapter, the author attempts to provide an overview of structural and physiological alterations in FD beyond those demonstrable by conventional tests used to separate organic dyspepsia from its functional counterpart.

2. Current definition of Functional Dyspepsia

According to Rome III criteria, FD must include one or more of the following symptoms: bothersome postprandial fullness, early satiation, epigastric pain and epigastric burning; with no evidence of structural disease, including use of upper gastrointestinal endoscopy, which is likely to explain the symptoms. Criteria should be fulfilled for at least 3 months with symptom onset at least 6 months previously [1].

Older terms that represent FD are non-ulcer dyspepsia, idiopathic or essential dyspepsia. The term non ulcer dyspepsia is still popular but no longer recommended because it implies that the patient has symptoms similar to peptic ulcer disease without having an actual ulcer on endoscopic examination. The spectrum of symptoms in FD includes epigastric pain syndrome and postprandial distress syndrome

At least 3 months, with onset at least 6 months previously, of one or more of the following:
• bothersome postprandial fullness • early satiation • epigastric pain • epigastric burning
AND
No evidence of structural disease (including upper endoscopy) that is likely to explain the symptoms.

Table 1. Rome III diagnostic criteria for functional dyspepsia [1]

3. Definitions of functional dyspepsia symptoms [1]

The Rome III committee proposed a distinction between meal-induced symptoms and meal-unrelated symptoms to be pathophysiologically, clinically and therapeutically relevant.

Epigastric pain syndrome:

1. Epigastric pain

Epigastric refers to the region between the umbilicus and lower end of the sternum, and marked by the midclavicular lines. Pain refers to a subjective, unpleasant sensation; some patients may feel that tissue damage is occurring.

2. Epigastric burning

Epigastric refers to the region between the umbilicus and lower end of the sternum, and marked by the midclavicular lines. Burning refers to an unpleasant subjective sensation of heat.

Postprandial distress syndrome:

1. **Postprandial fullness:** An unpleasant sensation like the prolonged persistence of food in the stomach.

2. **Early satiation:** A feeling that the stomach is overfilled soon after starting to eat, out of proportion to the size of the meal being eaten, so that the meal cannot be finished. Previously, the term 'early satiety' was used, but satiation is the correct term for the disappearance of the sensation of appetite during food ingestion.

Recent research findings indicate that postprandial distress syndrome and epigastric pain syndrome overlap in majority of patients with FD [11]. The implication of this is that the value of dividing FD into the subgroups of postprandial distress syndrome and epigastric pain syndrome is thus questionable [11]

4. Evaluating a patient with dyspepsia

4.1. Symptom-based diagnosis

The introduction of Rome criteria and Rome process was a milestone in the management of FGIDs. However, the high turnover of Rome criteria is a testimony to the fact that symptom-based diagnosis has limitations. Symptoms may be perceived differently within different cultures and languages. It has been recommended that the current Rome III questionnaire be translated into local languages [12]. Symptoms are poor predictors of FD and significant overlaps are often seen with functional disorders including functional heartburn and irritable bowel syndrome. [13-22].

One of the difficulties encountered in evaluating a patient with dyspepsia is that symptoms are nonspecific and cannot accurately differentiate an organic process from a functional disorder. Neither clinical impression, nor computer models incorporating patient demographics, risk factors, history items, and symptoms can distinguish between organic and functional disease in patients referred for endoscopic evaluation of dyspepsia([23].

There is also a high degree of overlap between FD symptoms and those of gastroparesis [1, 24-29]. In FD, the predominant sensation of early satiety was found to be closely associated with impaired accommodation, although it was also present in more than 30% of patients with delayed gastric emptying [26]. Nausea and vomiting, thought to be cardinal symptoms of gastroparesis, are present in at least 20-50% of patients with FD [25, 30, 31]. Epigastric pain thought to be a cardinal symptom of FD is also present in up to 90% of patients with gastroparesis (GP) [32, 33]. Generally, common symptoms of gastric neuromuscular dysfunction are nonspecific and cannot reliably predict the underlying pathophysiology [24-26, 34]. Furthermore, recent research data indicate that rapid gastric emptying has been implicated in functional dyspepsia symptoms, especially in the postprandial distress syndrome [35, 36]. Enhanced antral contractility, decreased duodenal feedback inhibition and impaired accommodation represent the underlying mechanisms [37, 38].

The current approach is to view functional dyspepsia and idiopathic gastroparesis, not as completely distinct disorders, but as a broad, continuous spectrum, with significant overlap. It has been proposed that these 2 entities be reclassified under the umbrella term of functional dyspepsia with or without disordered gastric emptying [39], to enable clinicians and researchers to focus on predominant symptoms expressed by the majority of patients with this disorder.

4.2. Age

Older age is an important predictor for the presence of organic disease. The American Gastroenterological Association recommends proceeding directly to endoscopy in patients older than 55 years [40], however, there has been debate about a lower cut-off age of 35 to 45 years in men [41]. The optimal age threshold for endoscopy is unclear but 55 years seems a reasonable cut-off because cancer is rare in younger patients but no age threshold is absolute [42] Age specific thresholds to trigger endoscopic evaluation may differ by sex and locality [43, 44] Prompt endoscopy in patients over 50 years regardless of alarm status has been shown to increase the proportion of curable cases of upper gastrointestinal malignancies by as much as 30% [45-47], but the cost-effectiveness of initial endoscopy in this age group for improving survival of cancer patients is uncertain [47, 48]. Distinct upper gastrointestinal malignancy incidence rates and various distributions of its topographical types in different populations [49-52], as well as differences in Helicobacter pylori infection rates [53, 54] could partly explain the variable results.

4.3. Alarm features

Alarm features include unintended weight loss, family history of upper gastrointestinal cancer, gastrointestinal bleeding, progressive dysphagia, odynophagia, unexplained iron deficiency anemia, persistent vomiting, palpable mass, lymphadenopathy and jaundice. These features are useful in identifying high risk patients who need early endoscopy. The absence of alarm features makes the likelihood of finding important structural causes for dyspepsia very low. However, a meta-analysis found that negative predictive value of alarm features was poor (6%) [55]. Worse still, subjects with organic pathologies may also have FD. [56]

4.4. Helicobacter pylori testing

Testing for Helicobacter pylori in dyspepsia may be used to select the subgroup of dyspeptic patients who have Helicobacter-related dyspepsia. The Asian consensus guideline posits that this is strictly not a form of FD. Proponents of this argue that gastritis can now be identified easily with advanced endoscopic techniques, and that Helicobacter pylori-dyspepsia is a form of post-infectious FD [2]. Exclusion of Helicobacter pylori infection should be an important part of diagnostic exercise in parts of the world where the burden of infection is high [2]. The effect of Helicobacter pylori eradication on the amelioration of symptoms in patients with FD has been evaluated in several large, well-designed, randomized controlled trials, but the results were conflicting [57-61]. Eradication of Helicobacter pylori in FD appears to improve dyspeptic symptoms more in the Chinese population than in Western populations [2]

4.5. Gastric accommodation and visceral hypersensitivity

The accommodation reflex is a vagally mediated volume response of the upper part of the stomach after a meal. After ingestion of food, the gastric fundus spontaneously dilates and begins to store food [62]. Impairment of this accommodation reflex is known to correlate well with dyspeptic symptoms especially early satiation [63, 64]. Enhanced perception of physiological signals arising from the stomach (visceral hypersensitivity) is considered a hallmark of functional gastrointestinal disorders including FD [65]. Such hypersensitivity can be reproduced acutely by different types of mechanical gastric distension [66, 67]. However, it has not been possible to conclusively identify the site and mechanisms underlying visceral hypersensitivity in FD.

Gastric barostat is gold standard for investigating gastric accommodation. It is however, invasive, time-consuming and uncomfortable to patients. Newer techniques include single photon emission computed tomography (SPECT) [64], 2- and 3- dimensional gastric ultrasound [68] and magnetic resonance imaging [69]. These are noninvasive but their high cost, sophistication and radiation exposure make them less attractive.

Drinking test is simpler [70]. It is based on the assumption that gastric volume is reduced with impaired accommodation and therefore limits the drinking volume. This test has been validated against the gastric barostat but the reproducibility is limited due to differences in types of drink and rates of drinking. In general these tests are poorly associated with dyspeptic symptoms and cannot predict a response to treatment in FD. Therefore they are not yet available for routine clinical use.

4.6. Gastric emptying

Gastroparesis is a syndrome characterized by delayed gastric emptying in absence of mechanical obstruction. Its causes include diabetes mellitus, post-surgical and idiopathic [71].

Delayed gastric emptying occurs in 23-59% of patients with FD [72]. Research has shown that delayed gastric emptying may be related to postprandial fullness and vomiting with symptoms being more frequently found in female patients than in males [73-75]. Other studies have failed to confirm any difference in the occurrence of FD symptoms between patients with normal or delayed gastric emptying [76, 77]

Assessment of gastric emptying is commonly performed for such indications as nausea, vomiting and dyspepsia. However, there is a poor correlation of symptoms to observed abnormalities.

Techniques of gastric emptying include scintigraphy, which is the standard method in clinical practice, but is associated with radiation exposure. Newer non-invasive methods include wireless motility capsule and gastric emptying breath testing. Ultrasound, single-photon emission computed tomography (SPECT) and magnetic resonance imaging (MRI) are predominantly research tools.

4.7. Chemical hypersensitivity test

The duodenum is implicated in the pathophysiology of FD. Duodenal hypersensitivity and abnormal responses to various substances have been observed in FD.

Duodenal hypersensitivity to lipid: Duodenal infusion of lipid in subjects with FD increased gastric distension and symptoms in a dose-dependent fashion [78]. Symptom relief is achieved with administration of Loxiglumide, a cholecystokinin A receptor antagonist and this suggests that cholecystokinin release following a lipid stimulus is the mediator of gastric hypersensitivity in FD [79] Using cholecystokinin infusion as a challenge test is appealing [80] but is not yet available for clinical use.

Buspirone challenge test [81] is another chemical hypersensitivity test. This chemical is a serotonin 1A agonist that acts at the hypothalamic level to stimulate prolactin release. The extent of prolactin release following Buspirone challenge is a reliable measure of central 5HT sensitivity which can be impaired in patients with FD [82, 83].

Duodenal sensitivity to acid infusion: Studies on the presence of duodenal hypersensitivity to acid in FD patients and its role in the pathophysiology of FD remain controversial. Samson et al [84] reported that duodenal acid infusion induced nausea in a subset of FD patients, but not in healthy controls, suggesting the presence of duodenal hypersensitivity to acid in FD patients. However, other studies found that dyspeptic symptoms such as nausea could be induced by duodenal acidification in healthy volunteers [85].

5. Empirical treatment

Therapeutic trial may be employed as a means of diagnosis. This has proved successful in the management of GERD but the story in FD is entirely different because its pathogenesis is poorly understood and there is no effective treatment. Also, there is often a substantial placebo effect.

http://dx.doi.org/10.5772/56620

The new drug, Acotiamide, an acetylcholinesterase inhibitor is promising and has been shown to be efficacious and safe in the elimination of meal-related FD symptoms [86]. Though not yet approved for treatment of FD, it holds high promise as no adverse events were recorded.

5.1. Duodenal eosinophilia

Eosinophils and mast cells may be specifically recruited to the duodenum, altering sensation and motility [87]. The duodenum, which is often ignored in the search for pathophysiologic explanations for FD may be key to the symptom experience in FD. Mast cells induce eosinophil migration and eosinophils activate mast cells [88]. Degranulation from mast cells and eosinophils leads to neural stimulation and smooth muscle contraction, which in turn results in gastrointestinal symptoms, such as abdominal pain and bloating [89]. While a significant increase in mast cells has not been observed in the duodenum of patients with FD, duodenal eosinophilia in FD has been described [90, 91]. This finding is exciting, because, in patients undergoing endoscopy, duodenal biopsy is safe and easy to perform. This finding also has a potential therapeutic implication which further research would unravel.

Putative test/Abnormality	Comments/Pitfalls
Helicobacter pylori testing	Useful in identifying patients who have Helicobacter pylori – associated dyspepsia
Gastric accommodation test	Several tests have been developed. Invasiveness, high cost, patient discomfort and radiation exposure remain challenges
Gastric emptying test	Scintigraphy is currently available for clinical use.
Empirical treatment	Not a viable option because of poorly understood pathogenesis and lack of effective treatment
Duodenal eosinophilia	Initial studies promising. Larger studies needed.
Duodenal acid infusion	Results controversial
Duodenal lipid infusion	Duodenal hypersensitivity to lipids consistently obtained from most studies
Chemical hypersensitivity tests	Several candidate chemicals at various stages of development

Table 2. Summary of structural and functional abnormalities of the gastrointestinal tract in functional dyspepsia

In conclusion, dyspepsia is a very common clinical problem globally. Majority of patients with this problem have FD, defined traditionally as dyspepsia in which investigations, including upper gastrointestinal endoscopy fail to reveal a structural, biochemical or other pathophysiologic reason for the symptom. The pathophysiology of FD remains poorly understood.

Recent information from research shows that there are structural and physiological changes in FD that may hold the key to further understanding of the pathogenesis of this disease. These include Helicobacter pylori infection, abnormalities of gastric accommodation, abnormalities of gastric emptying, duodenal eosinophilia duodenal hypersensitivity to acid and lipids. These changes have prospects of being deployed in future for the diagnostic evaluation of FD. The implication of this is that FD may not be idiopathic after all. Research is likely to shed more light on this in future.

Author details

Sylvester Chuks Nwokediuko[1,2*]

Address all correspondence to: scnwokediuko@yahoo.com

1 College of Medicine, University of Nigeria, Enugu Campus, Nigeria

2 University of Nigeria Teaching Hospital Ituku/Ozalla, Enugu, Nigeria

References

[1] Tack J, Talley NJ, Camilleri M, Holtmann G, Hu P, Malagelada J, et al. Functional gastroduodenal disorders. Gastroenterology. 2006;130:1466–1479.

[2] Miwa H, Ghoshal UC, Gonlachanvit S, Gwee KA, Ang TL, Chang FY et al. Asian Consensus Report on Functional Dyspepsia. J Neurogastroenterol Motil 2012; 18:150-168.

[3] El-Serag H.B., Talley N.J. Systemic review: The prevalence and clinical course of functional dyspepsia. Aliment Pharmacol Ther 2004; 19: 643–654

[4] Talley N.J., Silverstein M.D., Agreus L., Nyren O., Sonnenberg A., Holtmann G. AGA technical review: evaluation of dyspepsia. American Gastroenterological Association. Gastroenterology 1998; 114: 582–595.

[5] Jones, R.H. Approaches to uninvestigated dyspepsia. Gut 2002; 50(Suppl 4): iv42-iv46.

[6] Talley NJ, Koch KL, Koch M, Nyrem O, Stanghellini V. Functional dyspepsia: a classification with guidelines for diagnosis and management. Gastrointest Int 1991;4:145–160.

[7] Talley NJ, Axon A, Bytzer P, Holtmann G, Lam SK, Van Zanten S. Management of uninvestigated and functional dyspepsia: a Working Party Report for the World Congresses of Gastroenterology 1998. Aliment Pharmacol Ther 1999;13:1135-1148.

[8] Tally NJ, Stanghellini V, Heading RC, Koch KL, Malagelada JR, Tytgat GNJ. Functional gastroduodenal disorders. Gut 1999a; 45 (Suppl) II:37–42.

[9] Talley, N.J., Ruff, K., Jiang, X. and Jung, H.K. The Rome III classification of dyspepsia: will it help research? Dig Dis 2008; 26: 203_209.

[10] Talley NJ, Stanghellini V, Heading RC, Koch KL, Malagelada JR, Tytgat GNJ. Functional dyspepsia. Aliment Pharmacol Ther 2004; 19: 643-654.

[11] Vakil N, Halling K, Ohlsson L, Wernersson B. Symptom overlap between postprandial distress and epigastric pain syndromes of the Rome III dyspepsia classification. Am J Gastroenterol 2013; 108: 767-774

[12] Lee YY, Waid A, Tan HJ, Chua AS, Whitehead WE. The validity and reliability of the Malay-language translation of the Rome III Diagnostic Questionnaire for irritable bowel syndrome. J Gastroenterol Hepatol 2012;27:746-750.

[13] Kim JS, Lee KJ, Kim JH, Hahm KB, Cho SW. Functional gastrointestinal disorders in patients referred to specialist gastroenterologists in a tertiary hospital. Korean J Neurogastroenterol Motil 2004;10:111-117.

[14] Shah SS, Bhatia SJ, Mistry FP. Epidemiology of dyspepsia in the general population in Mumbai. Indian J Gastroenterol 2001;20: 103-106.

[15] Ghoshal UC, Abraham P, Bhatt C, Choudhuri G, Bhatia SJ, Shenoy KT et al. Epidemiological and clinical profile of irritable bowel syndrome in India: report of the Indian Society of Gastroenterology Task Force. Indian J Gastroenterol 2008;27:22-28.

[16] Okumura T, Tanno S, Ohhira M, Tanno S. Prevalence of functional dyspepsia in an outpatient clinic with primary care physicians in Japan. J Gastroenterol 2010;45:187-194.

[17] Hu WH, Wong WM, Lam CL, Lam KF, Hui WM, Lai KC et al. Anxiety but not depression determines health care-seeking behaviour in Chinese patients with dyspepsia and irritable bowel syndrome: a population-based study. Aliment Pharmacol Ther 2002;16:2081-2088.

[18] Hori K, Matsumoto T, Miwa H. Analysis of the gastrointestinal symptoms of uninvestigated dyspepsia and irritable bowel syndrome. Gut Liver 2009;3:192-196.

[19] Ghoshal UC, Singh R, Chang FY, Hou X, Wong BC, Kachintorn U. Epidemiology of uninvestigated and functional dyspepsia in Asia: facts and fiction. J Neurogastroenterol Motil 2011; 17: 235-244.

[20] Kitapçioğlu G, Mandiracioğlu A, Caymaz Bor C, Bor S. Overlap of symptoms of dyspepsia and gastroesophageal reflux in the community. Turk J Gastroenterol 2007;18:14-19.

[21] Lee SY, Lee KJ, Kim SJ, Cho SW. Prevalence and risk factors for overlaps between gastroesophageal reflux disease, dyspepsia, and irritable bowel syndrome: a population-based study. Digestion 2009;79: 196-201.

[22] Sperber AD. The challenge of cross-cultural, multi-national research : potential benefits in the functional gastrointestinal disorders. Neurogastroenterol Motil 2009;21:351-360.

[23] Moayyedi P, Talley NJ, Fennerty MB, Vakil N. Can the clinical history distinguish between organic and functional dyspepsia? JAMA 2006; 295:1566-1576.

[24] Parkman HP, Hasler WL, Fisher RS. American Gastroenterological Association technical review on the diagnosis and treatment of gastroparesis. Gastroenterology 2004; 127: 1592–622.

[25] Karamanolis G, Caenepeel P, Arts J., Tack J. Association of the predominant symptom with clinical characteristics and pathophysiological mechanisms in functional dyspepsia. Gastroenterology 2006; 130: 296–303.

[26] Van Lelyveld N, Schipper M, Samsom M. Lack of relationship between chronic upper abdominal symptoms and gastric function in functional dyspepsia. Dig Dis Sci 2008; 53: 1223–1230.

[27] Punkkinen J, Färkkilä M, Mätzke S, Korppi-Tommola T, Sane T, Piirilä P, Koskenpato J. Upper abdominal symptoms in patients with Type 1 diabetes: unrelated to impairment in gastric emptying caused by autonomic neuropathy. Diabet Med 2008; 25: 570–577.

[28] Abell TL, Bernstein RK, Cutts T, Farrugia G, Forster J, Hasler WL. Treatment of gastroparesis: a multidisciplinary clinicalreview. Neurogastroenterol Motil 2006; 18: 263–83.

[29] Cassilly DW, Wang YR, Friedenberg FK, Nelson DB, Maurer AH, Parkman HP. Symptoms of gastroparesis: use of the gastroparesis cardinal symptom index in symptomatic patients referred for gastric emptying scintigraphy. Digestion 2008; 78: 144–151.

[30] Tack J, Demedts I, Dehondt G, Caenepeel P, Fischler B, Zandecki M et al. Clinical and pathophysiological characteristics of acute-onset functional dyspepsia. Gastroenterology 2002; 122: 1738–1747.

[31] Bisschops R, Karamanolis G, Arts J, Caenepeel P, Verbeke K, Janssens J et al. Relationship between symptoms and ingestion of a meal in functional dyspepsia. Gut 2008; 57: 1495–1503

[32] Cherian D, Sachdeva P, Fisher RS Parkman HP. Abdominal pain is a frequent symptom of gastroparesis. Clin Gastroenterol Hepatol 2010; 8: 676–681.

[33] Hoogerwerf WA, Pasricha PA, Kalloo AN. Schuster MM. Pain: the overlooked symptom in gastroparesis. Am J Gastroenterol 1999; 94: 1029–1033.

[34] Fischler B, Vandenberghe J, Persoons P, Gucht VD, Broekaert D, Luyckx K et al. Evidence-based subtypes in functional dyspepsia with confirmatory factory analysis: psychosocial and physiopathological correlates. Gastroenterology 2001; 120(Suppl 1): A51-A52.

[35] Delgado-Aros S, Camilleri M, Cremonini F, Ferber I, Stephens D, Burton DD. Contributions of gastric volumes and gastric emptying to meal size and postmeal symptoms in functional dyspepsia. Gastroenterology 2004;127: 1685-1694.

[36] Kusano M, Zai H, Shimoyana Y, Hosaka H, Kuribayashi S, Kawamura O et al. Rapid gastric emptying, rather than delayed gastric emptying might provoke functional dyspepsia. J Gastroenterol Hepatol 2011; 26(Suppl 3): 75-78.

[37] Tack J, Bisschops R. Mechanisms underlying meal-induced symptoms in functional dyspepsia. Gastroenterology 2004; 127: 1844-1847.

[38] Bharucha AE, Manduca A, Lake DS, Fidler J, Edwards P, Grimm RC et al. Gastric motor disturbances in patients with idiopathic rapid gastric emptying. Neurogastroentero Motil 2011; 617-e252.

[39] Lacy BE. Functional dyspepsia and gastroparesis: one disease or two? Am J Gastroenterol 2012; 107: 1615-1620.

[40] Talley NJ. America Gastroenterological Association medical position statement: evaluation of dyspepsia. Gastroenterology 2005; 129: 1753-1755.

[41] Marmo R, Rotondano G, Piscopo R, Bianco MA, Russo P, Capobianco P et al. Combination of age and sex improves the ability to predict upper gastrointestinal malignancy in patients with uncomplicated dyspepsia: a prospective multicentre database study. Am J Gastroentero 2005; 100: 784-791.

[42] Canga C 3rd, Vakil N Upper gastrointestinal malignancy, uncomplicated dyspepsia, and the age threshold for early endoscopy. Am J Gastroenterol 2002; 97: 600-603

[43] Vakil N, Moayyedi P, Fennerty MB, Talley NJ. Limited value of alarm features in the diagnosis of upper gastrointestinal malignancy: systematic review and meta-analysis. Gastroenterology 2006; 131: 390-401.

[44] Lieberman D, Fennerty MB, Morris CD, Holub J, Eisen G, Sonnenberg A. Endoscopic evaluation of patients with dyspepsia: results from the national endoscopic data repository. Gastroenterology 2004; 127:1067-1075.

[45] Dickerson LM, King DE. Evaluation and management of nonulcer dyspepsia. Am Fam Physician 2004; 70: 107-114.

[46] Axon AT, Bell GD, Jones RH, Quine MA, McCloy RF. Guidelines on appropriate indications for upper gastrointestinal endoscopy. Working Party of the Joint Commit-

tee of the Royal College of Physicians of London, Royal College of of Surgeons of England, Royal college of Anaesthetists, Association of Surgeons, The British Society of Gastroenterology, and the Thoracic Society of Great Britain. BMJ 1995; 310: 853-856.

[47] Hallissey MT, Allum WH, Jewkes AJ, Ellis DJ, Fielding JW. Early detection of gastric cancer. BMJ 1990; 301: 513-515.

[48] Delaney BC, Wilson S, Roalfe A, Roberts L, Redman V, Wearn A et al. Cost effectiveness of initial endoscopy for dyspepsia in patients over age 50 years: a randomized controlled trial in primary care. Lancet 2000; 356: 1965-1969.

[49] Heikkinen M, Pikkarainen P, Takala J, Rasanen H, Julkunen R. Etiology of dyspepsia. Four hundred unselected consecutive patients in general practice. Scand J Gastroenterol 1995; 30: 519-523.

[50] Ayoola EA, al-Rashed RS, al-Moflesh IA, al-Faleh FZ, Laajam M. Diagnostic yield of upper gastrointestinal endoscopy in relation to age and gender: a study of 10112 patients. Hepatogastroenterology 1996; 43: 409-415.

[51] Mansi C, Mela GS, Pasini D, Grosso M, Corti L, Moretti M et al. Patterns of dyspepsia in patients with no clinical evidence of organic diseases. Dig Dis Sci 1990; 35: 1452-1458.

[52] Talley NJ. Nonulcer dyspepsia: current approaches to diagnosis and management. Am Fam Physician 1993, 47: 1407-1416.

[53] Ford AC, Axon AT. Epidemiology of Helicobacter pylori infection and public health implications. Helicobacter 2010; 15: 1-6.

[54] Babaei M, Pourfarzi F, Yazdanbod A, Chiniforash MM, Derakhshan MH, Mousavi SM et al. Gastric cancer in Ardabil, Iran- a review and update on cancer registry data. Asian Pac J Cancer Prev 2010; 11: 595-599.

[55] Fransen GA, Janssen MJ, Muris JW, Laheij RJ, Jansen JB. Meta-analysis: The diagnostic value of alarm symptoms for upper gastrointestinal malignancy. Aliment Pharmacol Ther 2004; 20: 1045-1052.

[56] Kinoshita Y, Chiba T; FUTURE Study Group. Characteristics of Japanese patients with chronic gastritis and comparison with functional dyspepsia defined by Rome III criteria: based on the large-scale survey, FUTURE study. Intern Med 2011;50:2269-2276.

[57] Kawamura A, Adachi K, Takashima T, Murao M, Katsube T, Yuki M et al. Prevalence of functional dyspepsia and its relationship with Helicobacter pylori infection in a Japanese population. J Gastroenterol Hepatol 2001; 16: 384-388.

[58] Moayyedi P, Soo S, Deeks J, Forman D, Mason J, Innes M et al. Systematic review and economic evaluation of Helicobacter pylori eradication treatment for non-ulcer dyspepsia. BMJ 2000; 321: 659-664.

[59] Laine L, Schoenfeld P, Fennerty MB. Therapy for Helicobacter pylori in patients with non-ulcer dyspepsia. A meta-analysis of randomized, controlled trials. Ann Intern Med 2001;134: 361-369.

[60] Miwa H, Hirai S, Nagahara A, Murai T, Nishira T, Kikuchi S et al. Cure of Helicobacter pylori infection does not improve symptoms in non-ulcer dyspepsia patients-a double- blind placebo-controlled study. Aliment Pharmacol Ther 2000; 14: 317-324.

[61] Wong QM, Xiao SD, Hu PJ, Wang WH, Gu Q, Huang JQ et al. Standard treatment for Helicobacter pylori infection is suboptimal in non-ulcer dyspepsia compared with duodenal ulcer in Chinese. Aliment Pharmaco Ther 2005; 21: 73-81.

[62] Aspiroz F, Melagelada JR. Physiological variations in canine gastric tone measured by an electronic barostat. Am J Physiol 1985; 248:G229-G237.

[63] Tack J, Piessevaux H, Coulie B, Caenepeel P, Janssens J. Role of impaired gastric accommodation to a meal in functional dyspepsia.Gastroenterology 1998;115:1346-1352.

[64] Piessevaux H, Tack J, Walrand S, Pauwels S, Geubel A. Intragastric distribution of a standardized meal in health and functional dyspepsia:correlation with specific symptoms. Neurogastroenterol Motil 2003;15:447-455.

[65] Aspiroz F, Bouin M, Camilleri M, Mayer EA, Poitras P, Serra J et al. mechanisms of hypersensitivity in IBS and functional disorders. Neurogastroenterol Motil 2007; 19:62-88.

[66] Camilleri M. Functional dyspepsia: mechanisms of symptom generation and appropriate management of patients. Gastroenterol Clin North Am 2007; 36: 649-664.

[67] Karamanolis G, Caenepeel P, Arts J, Tack J. Association of the predominant symptom with clinical characteristics and pathophysiological mechanisms in functional dyspepsia. Gastroenterology 2006; 130: 296-303.

[68] Van den Elzen BD, Bennink RJ, Wieringa RE, Tytgat GN, Boeckxstaens GE. Fundic accommodation assessed by SPECT scanning: comparison with the gastric barostat. Gut 2003;52:1548-1554.

[69] Mundt MW, Hausken T, Smout AJ, Samsom M. Relationships between gastric accommodation and gastrointestinal sensations in healthy volunteers. A study using the barostat technique and two- and three-dimensional ultrasonography. Dig Dis Sci 2005;50:1654-1660.

[70] Marciani L, Gowland PA, Spiller RC, Manoj P, Moore RJ, Young P et al. Effect of meal viscosity and nutrients on satiety, intra-gastric dilution, and emptying assessed by MRI. Am J Physiol Gastrointest Liver Physiol 2001;280:G1227-G1233.

[71] Soykan I, Sivri B, Sarosiek I, Kiernan B, McCallum RW. Demography, clinical characteristics, psychological and abuse profiles, treatment, and long-term follow-up of patients with gastroparesis. Dig Dis Sci 1998; 43: 2398-2404.

[72] Tack J, Bisschops R, Sarnelli G. Pathophysiology and treatment of functional dyspepsia. Gastroenterology 2004; 127: 1239-1255.

[73] Stanghellini V, Tosetti C, Paternico A, Barbara G, Morselli-Labate AM, Monetti N et al. Risk indicators of delayed gastric emptying of solids in patients with functional dyspepsia. Gastroenterology 1996; 110: 1036-1042.

[74] Tack J, Bisschops R. Mechanisms underlying meal-induced symptoms in functional dyspepsia. Gastroenterology 2004; 127: 1844-1847.

[75] Talley NJ, Locke GR 3rd, Lahr BD, Zeinsmeister AR, Tougas G, Liqozio G et al. Functional dyspepsia, delayed gastric emptying and impaired quality of life Gut 2006; 55: 933-939.

[76] Talley NJ, Verlinden M, Jones M. Can symptoms discriminate among those with delayed or normal gastric emptying in dysmotility-like dyspepsia? Am J Gastroenterol 2001; 96:1422-1428.

[77] Bredenoord AJ, Chial HJ, Camilleri M, Mullan BP, Murray JA. Gastric accommodation and emptying in evaluation of patients with upper gastrointestinal symptoms. Clin Gastroenterol Hepatol 2003; 1: 264-272.

[78] Feinle-Bisset C, Horowitz M. Dietary factors in functional dyspepsia. Neurogastroenterol Motil 2006;18:608-618.

[79] Chua AS, Bekkering M, Rovati LC, Keeling PW. Clinical efficacy and prokinetic effect of the CCK-A antagonist loxiglumide in nonulcer dyspepsia. Ann N Y Acad Sci 1994;713:451-453.

[80] Chua AS, Keeling PW. Cholecystokinin hyperresponsiveness in functional dyspepsia. World J Gastroenterol 2006; 12: 2688-2693.

[81] Chua AS, Keeling PW, Dinan TG. Role of cholecystokinin and central serotonergic receptors in functional dyspepsia. World J Gastroenterol 2006 ;12:1329-1335.

[82] Chua A, Keating J, Hamilton D, Keeling PW, Dinan TG. Central serotonin receptors and delayed gastric emptying in non-ulcer dyspepsia. BMJ 1992;305:280-282.

[83] Dinan TG, Mahmud N, Rathore O, Thakore J, Scott LV, Carr E et al. A double-blind placebo-controlled study of buspirone-stimulated prolactin release in non-ulcer dyspepsia-are central serotoninergic responses enhanced? Aliment Pharmacol Ther 2001;15:1613-1618.

[84] Samsom M, Verhagen MA, vanBerge Henegouwen GP, Smout AG. Abnormal clearance of exogenous acid and increased acid sensitivity of the proximal duodenum in dyspeptic patients. Gastroenterlogy 1999; 116: 515-520.

[85] di Stefano M, Vos R, Vanuytsel T, Janssens J, Tack J. Prolonged duodenal acid perfusion and dyspeptic symptom occurrence in healthy volunteers. Neurogastroenterl Motil 2009; 21: 712-e740.

[86] Matsueda K, Hongo M, Tack J, Saito Y, Kato H. A placebo-controlled trial of acotiamide for meal-related symptoms of functional dyspepsia. Gut 2012;61:821-828.

[87] Talley NJ, Walker MM, Aro P, Ronkainen J, Storskrubb T, Hindley LA et al. Non-ulcer dyspepsia and duodenal eosinophilia: an adult endoscopic population-based case-control study. Clin Gastroenterol Hepatol 2007, 5:1175-1183.

[88] Piliponsky AM, Pickholtz D, Gleich GJ, Levi-Schaffer F. Human eosinophils induce histamine release from antigen-activated rat peritoneal mast cells in late-phase allergic reactions. J Allergy Clin Immunol 2001;107: 993-1000.

[89] Powell N, Walker MM, Talley NJ. Gastrointestinal eosinophils in health, disease and functional disorders. Nat Rev Gastroenterol Hepatol 2010; 7: 146-156.

[90] Talley NJ, Walker MM, Aro P, Ronkainen J, Storskrubb T, Hindley LA et al. Non-ulcer dyspepsia and duodenal eosinophilia: an adult endoscopic population-based case-control study. Clin Gastroenterol Hepatol 2007; 5: 1175-1183.

[91] Walker MM, Talley NJ, Prasbhakar M, Pennaneac'h CJ, Aro P, Ronkainen J et al. Duodenal mastocytosis, eosinophilia and intraepithelial lymphocytosis as possible disease markers in the irritable bowel syndrome and functional dyspepsia. Aliment Pharmacol Ther 2009; 29: 765-773.

Chapter 3

Inflammation and the Biopsychosocial Model in Pediatric Dyspepsia

Jennifer Verrill Schurman and Craig A. Friesen

Additional information is available at the end of the chapter

http://dx.doi.org/10.5772/56635

1. Introduction

1.1. Diagnostic criteria

In the late 1980s, a group of experts met in Rome to establish symptom-based diagnostic criteria for functional gastrointestinal disorders (FGIDs). This first set of "Rome criteria," published in 1989, focused exclusively on adults [1]. In 1999, when these criteria were revised, a pediatric committee established a parallel set of diagnostic criteria for FGIDs in children and adolescents [2]. The Rome II pediatric subcommittee defined four pediatric disorders related to abdominal pain: functional dyspepsia (FD), irritable bowel syndrome (IBS), abdominal migraine, and functional abdominal pain. With Rome II, FD was defined as persistent or recurrent pain or discomfort centered in the upper abdomen (above the umbilicus) that was unrelated to a change in stool frequency or form and not exclusively relieved by defecation. Further, there had to be no evidence of an inflammatory, anatomic, metabolic, or neoplastic process to explain the patient's symptoms. Importantly, the committee determined that mild, chronic inflammatory changes on mucosal biopsies should not preclude the diagnosis of FD. Similar to the adult criteria on which they were based, the Rome II pediatric criteria for FD included 3 subtypes: 1) ulcer-like, in which pain was the predominant symptom; 2) dysmotility-like, in which discomfort (e.g., bloating, early satiety, postprandial fullness) was the predominant symptom; and, 3) unspecified.

In 2006, the same process of expert committees again revised the criteria, yielding the current Rome III criteria [3,4]. In adults, the previous FD subtypes were eliminated while two new subtypes were identified based on new studies generally utilizing factor analysis. The first subtype, postprandial distress syndrome, was defined as bothersome postprandial fullness occurring after ordinary sized meals and/or early satiation that prevents finishing a regular meal. The second subtype, epigastric pain syndrome, was defined as intermittent pain or burning localized to the epigastrium (i.e., not generalized or localized to other abdominal or chest regions) and of at least moderate severity. The Rome III pediatric subcommittee also eliminated the old subtypes, but did not adopt the new adult subtypes because of a lack of existing data to support their existence in children and adolescents. However, recent evidence suggests that the adult subtypes actually may have meaningful associations with mucosal inflammation and psychosocial functioning in pediatric FD [5].

1.2. Prevalence and presentation

Most pediatric gastroenterologists may not routinely use Rome criteria and differences exist in how the criteria are interpreted. Nevertheless, there is agreement that a strong majority of children with chronic abdominal pain presenting to pediatric gastroenterology practices fulfill criteria for an FGID, with the two most common being FD and IBS [6-9]. Community prevalence for FD is estimated at 3.5-27% in children/adolescents compared to 20-30% in adults [3,4].

In both pediatric and adult gastroenterology practices, FD frequently overlaps with IBS or gastroesophageal reflux [7,10]. Adult IBS overlap is associated with more psychological dysfunction including anxiety and depression, compared to "pure" FD, but this association does not appear to be present in pediatric overlap [11,12]. Pediatric FD is associated with lower quality of life, increased functional disability, and increased likelihood of meeting criteria for an anxiety disorder relative to healthy children [13]. In adults with FD, the association with anxiety appears to be specific to patients with postprandial distress syndrome, with this relationship also apparent in children/adolescents with symptoms consistent with postprandial distress syndrome [5,14].

1.3. Etiology

FD, like all FGIDs, is probably best understood through a biopsychosocial model (see Figure 1). This model states that symptoms are likely the result of varying contributions from, and interactions between, biological/physiological factors (e.g. inflammation, mechanical disturbances, hypersensitivity), psychological factors (e.g. anxiety, depression, somatization), and social factors (e.g. interactions with parents, teachers, or peers). Within this model, there is less emphasis on the "cause" of symptoms than on "contributors" to its emergence and maintenance. This model would suggest that there is value in identifying and targeting all of the factors which might be contributing to symptom generation in children with FD. It also would suggest that there is value in understanding the mechanisms by which the factors interact with one another, as these mechanisms represent additional opportunities for clinical intervention.

2. The role of inflammation in functional dyspepsia

Inflammation has the potential to contribute to the development of FGIDs via the release of specific mediators that impact mechanisms known to play a role in the pathogenesis of these conditions. Acute gastrointestinal inflammation and injury are associated with both peripheral

http://dx.doi.org/10.5772/56635

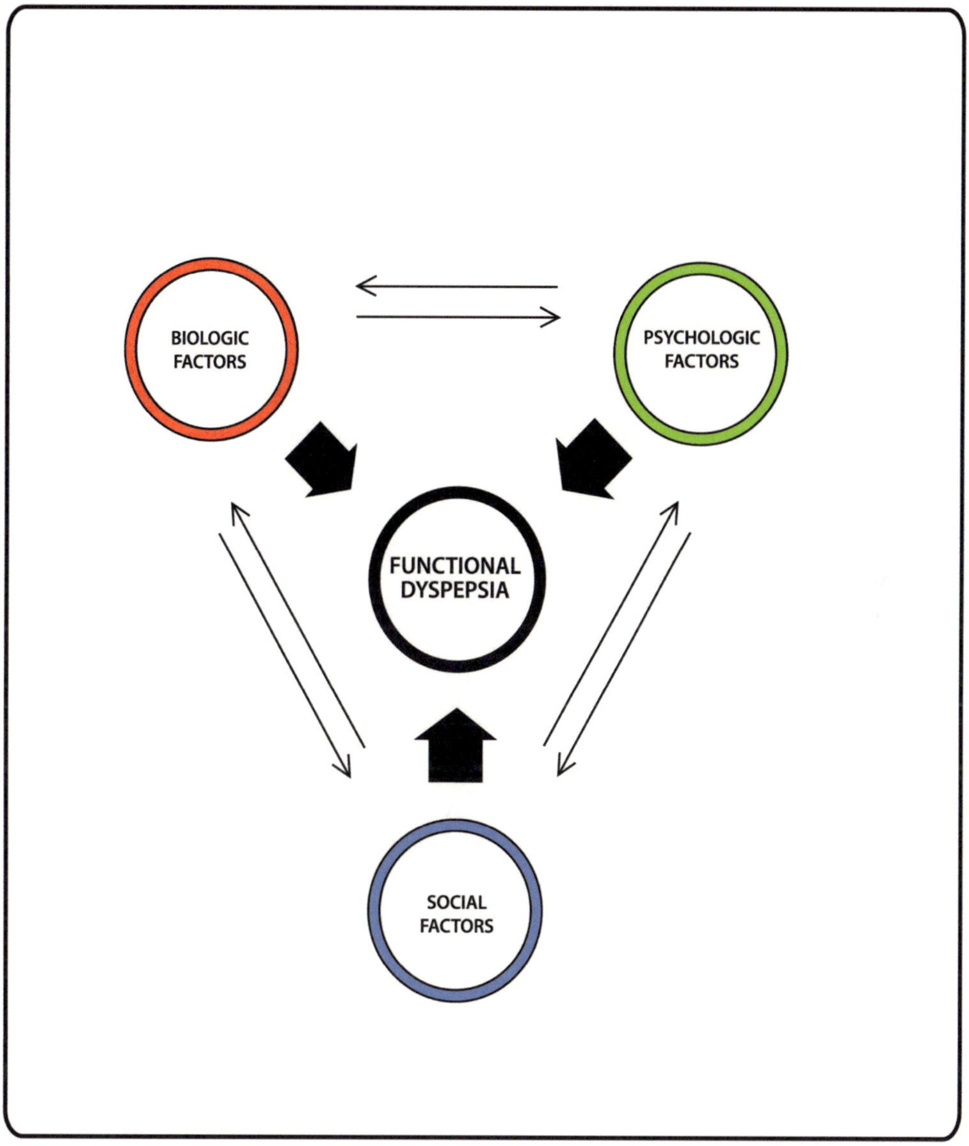

Figure 1. The Biopsychosocial Model of FD

and central sensitization of the nervous system, which results in visceral hyperalgesia [15]. Neuroplastic changes may occur that affect the response thresholds of enteric nerves, thereby negatively impacting both sensitivity and motility [16]. Both motility and sensitivity responses to acute inflammation in adults generally are reversible; however, animal model responses suggest that, if inflammation occurs in neonates, neuroplastic changes and sensitivity may persist into adulthood [17,18]. Visceral sensitization may be even more relevant in instances where there is chronic inflammation with ongoing mediator release, as there may be subsequent effects on visceral sensitivity that compound and prolong the issue.

The role of inflammation in FD has historically been controversial. However, emerging evidence supports its role as a contributing factor in the biopsychosocial model of FD. In fact, inflammation may be of particular importance in this model, as it interacts with a number of other factors and may actually mediate the relationship between psychologic and physiologic factors. The remainder of this chapter focuses on examination of inflammation within the biopsychosocial model of FD, laying out the current evidence for its prevalence, mechanisms of action, relationship with other important factors, and implications for evaluation and treatment.

2.1. Chronic inflammation

Upper endoscopy is commonly performed in children with chronic abdominal pain in general and children with functional dyspepsia in particular. Histologic inflammation is common in these patients. In children with chronic abdominal pain, esophagitis is common and would implicate gastroesophageal reflux as a contributor or cause of pain [19]. In one study of children with FD, specifically, histologic esophagitis was found in 18%, gastritis in 21%, and duodenitis in 13% [10]. Higher prevalences for gastritis, ranging from 43% to 71%, have been reported by others [20,21]. For the broader group of children with chronic abdominal pain, histologic inflammation has been documented in up to 79%, with an increase in mononuclear cells (indicative of chronic inflammation) in the antrum of 55% and in the duodenum of 16% of these children [19].

Most of these patients have chronic inflammation of which the clinical significance is unknown. Chronic gastritis is not associated with electrogastrographic abnormalities, delayed gastric emptying, or psychologic dysfunction in children with FD [5,22]. Despite this, chronic active gastritis (manifest as lymphocytic and neutrophilic inflammation) has been associated with a higher prevalence of nocturnal pain [21]. Chronic gastritis has been associated with an increased prevalence of postprandial pain [5].

2.2. Mast cells

Increased mucosal mast cell density has been demonstrated in the gastric corpus and antrum in adults with FD [23,24]. In adults with gastritis, mast cell density is significantly increased and generally correlates with the intensity of the inflammation [25]. Though findings have been variable, increased mast cell density appears isolated to the stomach in adults with FD; increased duodenal mast cell density is more associated with IBS [24,26]. In addition, increased mast cells in the proximal stomach in adults with FD have been associated with hypersensitivity; these mast cells will degranulate with balloon distension of the proximal stomach [27].

Due to a lack of normal control data, it is not known if gastric mast cells are elevated in pediatric FD. However, antral mast cells do appear to be actively degranulating in children with FD, with a mean degranulation index of 67% and greater than 50% degranulation in over 80% of patients [28]. In children with FD, mast cell density positively correlates with slower gastric emptying and increased gastric dysrhythmia (primarily preprandial bradycardia) in children with FD [28]. Further, this dysrhythmia is associated with increased postprandial pain [29].

2.3. Eosinophils

Ethical considerations preclude undertaking studies that assess eosinophil density in healthy pediatric controls. However, the available pediatric literature indicates that it is reasonable to consider eosinophil densities ≥10/hpf in the antrum and >20/hpf in the duodenum to be abnormal. In a pediatric autopsy study, eosinophil density was <10/hpf in the antrum of all subjects and ≤20/hpf in the duodenum of 82%, even though symptoms could not be documented [30]. Another study reviewed biopsies from 682 presumably symptomatic children referred for endoscopy, documenting eosinophil density ≤10/hpf in the antrum in 90% and ≤20/hpf in the duodenum in 93% [31].

While certain cut-off points for density seem reasonable, eosinophil density may not be completely informative. Eosinophil biologic activity occurs through mediator release or degranulation, and the effects are generally concentration-dependent. Important to consider is the fact that density and activation are not correlated events [32]. In one study involving 20 children with FD, eosinophil density >20/hpf was present in only 15%; however, moderate to extensive degranulation was demonstrated by electron microscopy in 95% [33].

Adult population studies have demonstrated increased duodenal eosinophil density in those with dyspepsia compared to controls, whereas antral eosinophils did not differ between the groups [34,35]. Higher eosinophil density and a higher prevalence of duodenal eosinophilia (as defined by application of the cut points outlined above) have been specifically associated with the postprandial distress syndrome subtype of FD in adults [36]. Duodenal biopsies from adults with FD also have revealed more extensive degranulation, including documentation of extracellular major basic protein; this corresponds to a similar finding of degranulation and release of major basic protein previously demonstrated in pediatric patients with FD [33,35].

Although no information is available for healthy children, tissue eosinophilia has been evaluated in the broad group of children with chronic abdominal pain, which provides some limited basis for comparison. In a study of 1191 children with chronic abdominal pain, eosinophilia was identified in the antrum or duodenum in 11.4% [37]. In another study, gastric eosinophilia was reported in 19% and duodenal eosinophilia in 32% of children with unspecified chronic abdominal pain [19]. In contrast, duodenal eosinophilia has been demonstrated in 79% of children specifically fulfilling FD criteria [38].

Antral eosinophil density does not appear to have any direct relationship to gastric electromechanical function in children with FD [28]. However, in patients with elevated mucosal eosinophils, antral CD3+ cell density does correlate with preprandial tachygastria, indicating that it may result from the interaction between different cell types [28].

3. Specific Conditions Associated with Mucosal Inflammation

There are a number of triggers or inciting events which may initiate an inflammatory response in the gastrointestinal tract, particularly with regard to recruitment and activation of mast cells and eosinophils. These include stress/anxiety, infection (including H. pylori), and allergy, as detailed below.

3.1. Stress/Anxiety

The involvement of inflammation in the biopsychosocial model is best illustrated by examining the stress response. Corticotropin releasing hormone (CRH), produced by the hypothalamus (as well as immune cells including lymphocytes and mast cells) is a major mediator of the stress response in the hypothalamic-pituitary-adrenal axis and, subsequently, within the brain-gut axis. CRH has central nervous system (CNS) effects which may alter central processing of nociceptive messages, leading to anxiogenic and depressive effects. The stress response also results in physiologic effects which may be relevant to FGIDs, including inflammation and alterations of sensorimotor function such as altered gastric accommodation, gastric dysmotility, and visceral hypersensitivity.

The relationship between the CNS and gastrointestinal pathophysiology appears bidirectional. In a rodent model, gastric irritation in the neonatal period induces a long lasting increase in depression- and anxiety-like behaviors. This, in turn, is associated with an increased expression of CRH in the hypothalamus and increased sensitivity of the hypothalamic-pituitary-adrenal axis to stress [39]. CRH stress systems may be activated by afferent nerves from inflamed sites or via cytokines including TNF-α, IL-1, IL-6, and IL-12 [40]. The majority of studies support an enhanced hypothalamic-pituitary-adrenal axis in at least some adults with IBS, although results have been variable [41-45].

Corticotropin releasing hormone receptors are widely expressed including within the gastrointestinal tract and immune cells. Mast cells express both CRH1 and CRH2 receptor subtypes at their surface [46]. Most of the inflammatory cell actions, including those on mast cells, occur via CRH2 receptors. Once mast cells are activated, they release mediators which recruit and activate eosinophils. Both of these cell types are interactive in a bi-directional fashion with T helper cells (Th; see Figure 2).

In addition to this indirect pathway, there also may be a direct effect for CRH on eosinophils. In a rodent model, psychologic stress results in eosinophils expressing CRH [47]. CRH is not expressed on eosinophils in the intestines of the mice except under psychologic stress and decreases after the stress is removed, with the reversion requiring longer periods of time as the length of the stressor increases [47]. A high correlation exists between anxiety scores and mucosal eosinophil density in children with FD [48]. Antral mast cell density also correlates with anxiety scores in children with FD [5]. Stress appears to shift the relative proportion and trafficking of T helper lymphocytes towards a Th2 or "allergic" phenotype [40]. This shift is driven by central and peripheral CRH, catecholamines, and histamine via H2 receptors. The Th2 phenotype is associated with release of IL-4, IL-10, and IL-13, which stimulate growth and activation of mast cells and eosinophils [40]. Shifting from a Th1 to a Th2 response may be the mechanism through which low grade inflammation leads to visceral sensitivity and motility disturbances; eosinophils and mast cells represent the key effector cells [49].

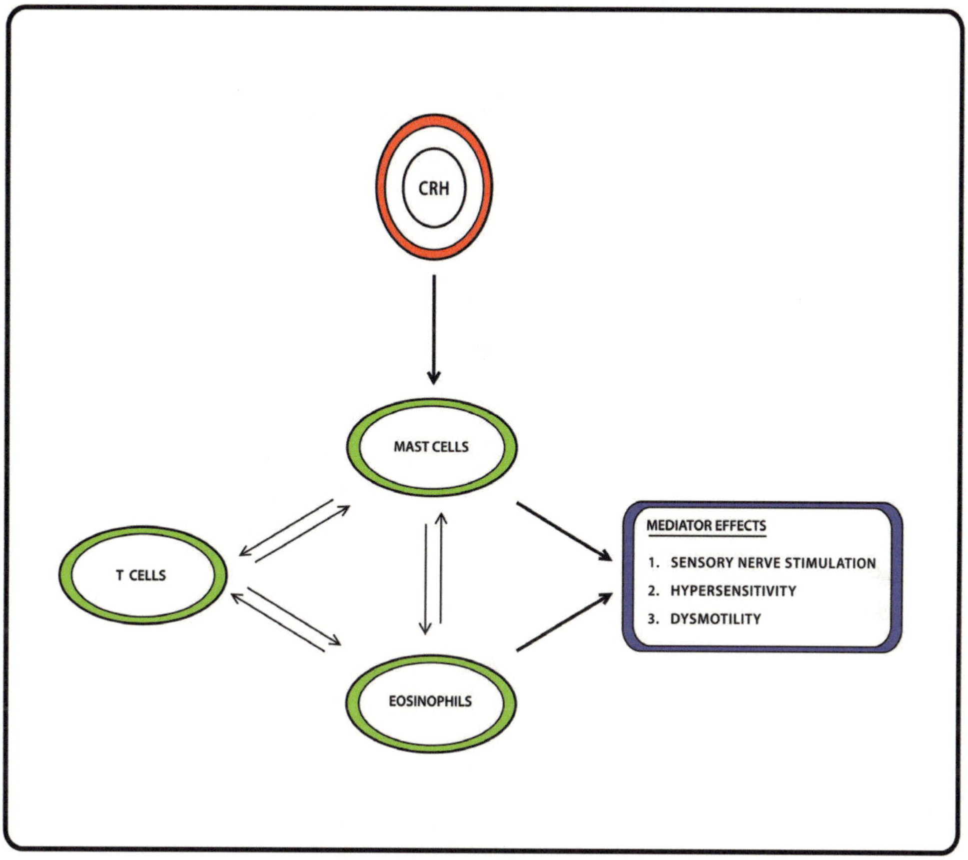

Figure 2. The Relationship between CRH Activation and Inflammatory Cells in FD Symptom Generation

Once activated by CRH, mast cells may release pre-formed and newly synthesized cytokines, including interleukins (IL-4, IL-5, IL-6) and tumor necrosis factor (TNF-α) among others [50,51]. In adults, there is selective luminal release of tryptase and histamine from jejunal mast cells under cold stress; the magnitude of release is similar to that induced by antigen exposure in food allergic patients [52]. Once released, mast cell and eosinophil mediators can stimulate afferent nerves sending a "pain" message, sensitize afferent nerves resulting in visceral hypersensitivity, and alter electromechanical function (see Figure 2). Histamine also can stimulate afferent sensory nerves via H2 receptors [53]. Consistent with this, experimental anxiety decreases gastric compliance and accommodation and increases epigastric symptom scores during a standard nutrient challenge [54].

3.2. Infection

FD has been reported at a higher prevalence following both bacterial and parasitic infections [55]. It seems likely that FD may also be induced by viral gastroenteritis similar to what has been reported with IBS. In a large cohort of adults that were evaluated 8 years after bacterial dysentery, an increased prevalence of FD was found compared to non-infected controls [56]. Consistent with the biopsychosocial model, anxiety and depression were independent risk factors for developing post-infectious FD [56]. In another study, 82 adults were identified with persistent abdominal symptoms following *Giardia* infection; 24.3% of these met criteria for FD, while 80.5% met criteria for IBS [57]. Over half of these patients reported exacerbation due to specific foods and nearly half reported exacerbations with physical or mental stress [57]. Rates of post-infectious FD appear similar in pediatric populations. In a study of 88 children with a previous positive bacterial stool culture, FD was present in 24% and IBS in 87% [58]. Fifty-six percent of these patients reported the onset of abdominal pain after the acute infection.

Post-infectious FD appears to represent an impaired ability to terminate the inflammatory response after the offending pathogen has been eliminated, but also may involve neuroplastic changes in visceral and central afferent pathways as it is associated with impaired accommodation and increased sensitivity to distension [59-61]. Post-infectious FD patients frequently demonstrate histologic duodenitis, with a severe grade in 57% [62]. Post-infectious FD is associated with increased macrophages and may be associated with increased CD8+ cells [62, 63]. Findings regarding CD8+ cells however have been variable [62,63]. Duodenal eosinophilia has also been described in post-infectious FD [49]. In addition, gastric mast cells are significantly increased in post-infectious FD as compared to healthy controls [64]. Post-infectious FD is associated with increased gastric release of histamine and 5HT, as well as increased number of mast cells within 5 μm of nerve fibers as compared to healthy controls or patients with FD that is not post-infectious [64].

H. pylori. The role of Helicobacter pylori (H. pylori) in FD remains incompletely defined and, as such, deserves particular attention within the scope of infectious organisms. Given that most people never demonstrate symptoms at all when colonized with H. pylori, it is possible that H. pylori has little to no contributory value for a significant subset of the population with FD. However, it is possible that H. pylori may generate symptoms as a primary chronic infection or, alternatively, patients may experience post-infectious FD once H. pylori has cleared in the much the same way as seen in other bacterial and parasitic infections.

Several studies have demonstrated efficacy in reducing FD symptoms with H. pylori eradication; however, others have found only a moderate (but statistically significant) effect or no clinical benefit to eradication at all [65-69]. A Cochrane review concluded that eradication was significantly better than placebo [69]. Response rates may be dependent on the specific symptom. For example, one study documented a positive response to H. pylori eradication, but only for the symptoms of epigastric pain and burning, indicating that efficacy may be restricted to patients with the epigastric pain syndrome subtype of FD [67]. A large number of patients with FD continue to experience symptoms following H. pylori eradication. These may be patients in whom H. pylori had no pathologic role, or may represent a group of patients who should be classified as post-infectious FD given that complete resolution of submucosal inflammation requires a prolonged period [70].

H. pylori colonization is generally associated with gastric and duodenal histologic inflammation. Histologic duodenitis has been associated with more severe symptoms when histologic gastritis also is present [71]. However, this finding has not been consistent, with others actually reporting an inverse relation between severity of symptoms and gastric inflammation [72]. H. pylori colonization in children is associated with increased mucosal lymphocytes, plasma cells, neutrophils, and eosinophils, which decrease with eradication [20]. H. pylori colonization may also be associated with increased antral mast cell density, though this may be H. pylori strain specific [73]. In the setting of nodular gastritis associated with HP colonization, eosinophils may be of particular significance. Nodularity is associated with the presence and density of eosinophils [74]. Patients with nodular gastritis have a higher incidence of FD symptoms which resolve with eradication therapy and improvement of gross endoscopic appearance [70]. Even in the absence of nodularity, H. pylori colonization is associated with increased antral eosinophils, as well as increased gastric fluid eosinophil cationic protein indicating eosinophilic activation [20,75,76]. These findings suggest a possible pathophysiologic role for eosinophils in contributing to symptoms in patients with H. pylori colonization or possibly following eradication.

Similar to post-infectious FD, H. pylori may be associated with electromechanical dysfunction which, in turn, can contribute to FD symptom generation. Though studies are conflicting, H. pylori has not consistently been associated with delayed gastric emptying or visceral hypersensitivity [77]. However, treatment with a prokinetic was found to be as effective as eradication at 12 months [78]. H. pylori also has been associated with an abnormal electrogastrogram that normalized in 83% with eradication [79]. H. pylori does not appear to have any effect on accommodation [60].

3.3. Allergy

The role of allergy in the development of FD has not been greatly studied. However, allergy may be important given the observed increases in, and activation of, mast cells and eosinophils in FD. FGIDs occur more commonly in children with a history of cow's milk allergy as infants [80]. In children with FD in association with cow's milk allergy, mucosal application of cow's milk is associated with increased eosinophils and mast cells, as well as rapid degranulation, within 10 minutes of application [81]. In addition, cow's milk exposure is associated with increased mast cells within 5 μm of nerves [81]. Adult FD patients with a history of allergy have increased duodenal eosinophil density [36]. In addition, lymphoid hyperplasia is significantly more frequent in children with abdominal pain associated with food allergies [19]. Lymphoid hyperplasia is associated with food hypersensitivity although this reaction may be local reactivity only as it is associated with normal skin prick tests and normal serum IgE levels [82,83].

Food allergy, similar to post infectious FD and H. pylori colonization, also may cause electromechanical dysfunction. Exposure to cow's milk in allergic FD children resulted in increased bradygastria [81]. In infants with cow's milk allergy, exposure results in gastric arrhythmias and delayed gastric emptying [84].

Whether food allergy accounts for a substantial portion of children with FD is not clear. One study found no significant increase in immunoreactivity to common food allergens in FD children with duodenal eosinophilia, although it is possible that the reaction was localized to the mucosa [85]. It is also possible that environmental allergens may be playing a role. Antigen exposure in adults with birch pollen allergy results in an increase in mucosal major basic protein positive eosinophils and IgE-bearing cells, as well as in FD symptoms, in the majority of patients [86]. Information in this area remains quite limited.

4. Implications for Care

4.1. Evaluation

The current approach to the pediatric FD patient has not been thoroughly studied. Based on existing small studies in children and large studies in adults, however, it appears reasonable to treat empirically with acid reducing medications and proceed with endoscopy with biopsies for non-responders. There may be value in evaluating mucosal biopsies for eosinophil density, particularly those obtained from the duodenum. A reasonable standard would be to consider antral eosinophil density >10/hpf and duodenal eosinophil density >20/hpf as abnormal. Despite current information implicating a role for mucosal mast cells, particularly in the antrum, it is less clear if there is value in determining mast cell density. The latter would require special immunohistochemical stains and the standard for normal is even less well defined than for eosinophils.

4.2. Treatment

Medications targeting mast cells or eosinophils could offer benefit by decreasing either cell density or activation. Such agents include corticosteroids and mast cell stabilizers. In addition, medications potentially could provide relief by targeting receptors for specific mediators once released by either cell. Although there is no current means for identifying the specific mediators generating symptoms in a particular patient, antagonists are available for some mediators, such as histamine, cysteinyl leukotrienes, and TNF- α. Finally, other treatments exist that may provide relief by targeting other factors, such as CRH, that may play an important role in activation and/or maintenance of inflammation. Consistent with a biopsychosocial model, combining treatments that address inflammation from different perspectives ultimately should be most beneficial.

Corticosteroids. Corticosteroids have not been evaluated in treating FD, but are commonly used in the treatment of eosinophilic gastroenteritis, although there are no placebo-controlled studies evaluating efficacy. The extensive side effect profile represents a significant draw back in considering their use long term. Budesonide may represent a safer alternative. Budesonide is a synthetic corticosteroid with high topical activity and substantial first pass elimination, limiting systemic exposure [87]. The literature regarding budesonide and eosinophilic gastroenteritis is limited, consisting of only case reports where budesonide therapy has been reported to be effective against eosinophilia in the duodenum and jejunum [88-90].

Mast Cell Stabilizers. Mast cell stabilizers, including cromolyn and ketotifen, would represent an attractive potential therapy given data implicating mast cells in the generation of FD symptoms as previously discussed. These agents would have the potential to prevent release

http://dx.doi.org/10.5772/56635

of a variety of mediators with downstream effects. In one open-label observational study of children with FD in association duodenal eosinophilia, resolution of pain was demonstrated with use of oral cromolyn in 89% of patients who had previously failed to respond to H2 and combined H1/H2 antagonism [91]. There have been no other pediatric or adult studies on the use of mast cell stabilizers in patients with FD. Benefit has been demonstrated in adults with IBS and may be related to blocking allergic or immunologic reactions to foods [92-94]. Ketotifen, specifically, has been shown to significantly decrease pain in adults with IBS and to increase the threshold for discomfort in patients with visceral hypersensitivity [95]. Ketotifen also acts as an H1 antagonist, so the effects may not be directly, or completely, related to mast cell stabilization.

Antihistamine Medications and Proton Pump Inhibitors (PPI). Acid reduction remains the most common treatment prescribed empirically by pediatric gastroenterologists for children with FD [9]. While there are numerous adult studies to support this practice, pediatric studies are limited. In children with chronic abdominal pain, famotidine (H2 recptor antagonist - H2RA) was superior to placebo in global improvement, with clear benefit to those with FD [96]. In a large pediatric study, omeperazole was shown to have a very modest advantage in the relief of all symptoms as compared to either famotidine or ranitidine; however, there was no significant difference between the three with regard to resolution of abdominal pain, epigastric pain, nausea, or vomiting specifically [97].

In adults, H2 antagonism has been shown to improve at least some symptoms associated with FD, including abdominal pain, indigestion, belching, and gastroesophageal reflux symptoms [98,99]. H2 antagonists have been shown to be superior to prokinetic medications and short term use of an anxiolytic [100,101]. A meta-analysis evaluating the use of PPIs in adult FD determined that they were superior to placebo in symptom reduction [102]. Studies of omeperazole, lansoprazole, and pantoprazole have demonstrated a modest superiority to placebo in symptom reduction which is limited to patients with ulcer-like or reflux-like FD [103-105]. Whether PPIs are superior to H2 antagonism is not completely clear. Omeperazole was found to have a modest increase in efficacy as compared to ranitidine at 4 weeks (51% vs. 36%), but there was no additional benefit at 6 months [101].

Given the response to PPIs, it would appear that at least some of the clinical improvement from H2 antagonism or PPIs is related directly to acid suppression. A significant portion of responders may derive benefit from treatment of overlap GERD, or possibly from peptic gastritis or duodenitis. Conversely, the benefit may be due to removing exposure to acid in patients with acid hypersensitivity. PPIs do not appear to have other benefits with regard to gastric emptying or myoelectrical function [106].

The benefit of H2 antagonism may be unrelated to acid reduction, at least in part. Histamine has direct gastric myogenic actions, modulates afferent enteric nerve excitability, and acts as an immunomodulating agent [53,107-111]. There may be additional benefit from H1 antagonism, as well. Combining an H1 antagonist with an H2 antagonist has been reported to relieve symptoms in 50% of children with FD associated with duodenal eosinophilia and in 79% of adults with FD associated with increased antral mast cell density who had previously failed to respond to acid reduction therapy [91,112]. H1 receptors affect smooth muscle contraction and visceral sensitivity [53]. In addition, some benefit from H1 antagonism may be due to an anxiolytic effect [113].

Cysteinyl Leukotriene (cysLT) Antagosists. CysLTs are another potential therapeutic target. The pattern of eosinophil degranulation in pediatric FD is consistent with the release of major basic protein, which is known to enhance the synthesis of cysLT; cysLT, in turn, stimulates smooth muscle contraction and recruitment of eosinophils [114]. CysLTs have been shown to alter mast cell function. CysLTs can induce IL-5 and TNF-α production in primed mast cells, an effect blocked by cysLT inhibition [115]. Leukotrienes (LTs) have the potential to increase intestinal sensory nerve sensitivity during inflammation. CysLTs have been shown to stimulate enteric neurons and to have a pro-contactile effect on the esophagus, stomach, small intestine, colon, and gallbladder [116-123].

Montelukast, a cysLT receptor antagonist, was superior to placebo with regard to relief of pain in a double-blind, placebo-controlled, cross-over trial of children with FD associated with duodenal eosinophilia [124]. The response rate was 84% in patients with eosinophil densities between 20 and 29/hpf versus 42% receiving placebo. A second study confirmed this high response rate [125]. In the latter study, the short term clinical response did not result from a decrease in eosinophil density or activation. This suggests that the effect of montelukast may be mediated through an enteric nerve effect on motility or sensitivity, something that remains to be demonstrated.

Anti-TNF-α. TNF-α would represent another potential therapeutic target. Mast cells are an important source of intestinal mucosal TNF-α in humans. CysLTs induce TNF-α production. TNF-α can recruit and prolong survival of eosinophils, as well promote a Th2 response depending on other chemokines present in the microenvironment [126-128]. Serum TNF-α concentration prior to treatment correlates negatively with the subsequent clinical response to montelukast in pediatric FD associated with duodenal eosinophilia, indicating that TNF-α may represent an alternative pathway for symptom generation in these patients. Although there are no controlled studies, anti-TNF-α has been reported to be effective in a series of children with resistant eosinophil disease, including patients with FD [129].

Biofeedback-Assisted Relaxation Training. The biopsychosocial model and CRH physiology would suggest a potential role for CRH antagonism or for controlling CRH secretion by controlling anxiety and the stress response. There are no previous studies evaluating CRH-antagonists in FD. Stress management would have the potential to control CRH secretion and, thereby, decrease inflammation. Biofeedback is a technique where individuals are trained to relieve physical or emotional symptoms using signals from their bodies that are displayed visually or aurally. It can be paired with relaxation training to yield biofeedback-assisted relaxation training. Biofeedback-assisted relaxation training may be considered as a solo therapy or, consistent with the biopsychosocial model, a stronger effect may occur in combining relaxation with medications targeting biologic factors such as inflammation. The combination of biofeedback-assisted relaxation training and fiber is superior to fiber alone in children with non-specific abdominal pain [130]. The effect of biofeedback-assisted relaxation training on inflammation has not been studied directly, but biofeedback-assisted relaxation training has been studied as adjunctive treatment in children with FD in association with duodenal

http://dx.doi.org/10.5772/56635

eosinophilia [131]. Children receiving medication plus biofeedback-assisted relaxation training demonstrated better outcomes with regard to pain intensity, duration of pain episodes, and global clinical improvement as compared to children receiving medications alone [131].

5. Conclusions

Current evidence implicates inflammation, particularly mast cells and eosinophils, in the pathophysiology of FD. FD in adults is associated with an increase in antral mast cell density and an increase in duodenal eosinophil density; elevated duodenal eosinophil density is frequently present in children with FD. Active degranulation of both cell types in children with FD suggests a pathophysiologic role. In children with FD, higher antral mast cell density is associated with gastric electromechanical dysfunction, psychologic dysfunction, and symptoms consistent with the postprandial distress syndrome subtype of FD defined for adults. Duodenal eosinophil density appears associated with anxiety in children with FD, but relationships with electromechanical dysfunction appear less direct. Both mast cells and eosinophils may have key roles in conditions that are associated with FD, including anxiety, infection (including H. pylori), and allergy. Ultimately, inflammation appears to be of particular importance in FD. Inflammation interacts with a number of other factors and may even mediate the relationship between psychologic and physiologic factors.

There may be efficacy in utilizing medications directed at inflammation, particularly mast cells and eosinophils. Most reports on treatment response consist of case series using H1/H2 antagonists, mast cell stabilizers, and anti-TNF-α. Consistent with a biopsychosocial model, some evidence exists to suggest that combining treatments targeting different components of the model that may influence inflammation can increase rates of symptom resolution in pediatric FD. There remains a need for placebo-controlled trials of the various medications and other treatments targeting inflammation which have been suggested to have efficacy, both alone and in thoughtful combination. Treatment for pediatric FD must continue to evolve if we are to prevent the significant downstream costs to the individual and society and, in this goal, inflammation appears an important primary target.

Author details

Jennifer Verrill Schurman[1] and Craig A. Friesen[2]

1 Division of Developmental & Behavioral Sciences, The Children's Mercy Hospitals & Clinics, Kansas City, MO, USA

2 Division of Gastroenterology, Hepatology, & Nutrition, The Children's Mercy Hospitals & Clinics, Kansas City, MO, USA

References

[1] Barbara L, Camilleri M, Corinaldesi R, Crean GP, Heading RC, Johnson AG, Malagelada JR, Stanghellini V, Wienbeck M. Definition and investigation of dyspepsia. Consensus of an international ad hoc working party. Dig Dis Sci 1989; 34: 1272-1276.

[2] Rasquin-Weber A, Hyman PE, Cucchiara S, Fleisher DR, Hyams JS, Milla PJ, Staiano A. Childhood functional gastrointestinal disorders. Gut 1999; 45:60-68.

[3] Rasquin A, Di Lorenzo C, Forbes D, Guiraldes E, Hyams JS, Staiano A, Walker LS. Childhood functional gastrointestinal disorders: Child/adolescent. Gastroenterology 2006; 130: 1527-1537.

[4] Tack J, Talley NJ, Camilleri M, Holtmann G, Hu P, Malagelada J-R, Stanghellini V. Functional gastroduodenal disorders. Gastroenterology 2006; 130: 1466-1479.

[5] Schurman JV, Singh M, Singh V, Neilan N, Friesen CA. Symptoms and subtypes in pediatric functional dyspepsia: Relation to mucosal inflammation and psychological functioning. J Pediatr Gastroenterol Nutr 2010; 51: 298-303.

[6] Walker LS, Lipani TA, Greene JW, Caines K, Stutts J, Polk DB, Caplan A, Rasquin-Weber A. Recurrent abdominal pain: Symptom subtypes based on Rome II criteria fro functional gastrointestinal disorders. J Pediatr Gastroenterol Nutr 2004; 38: 187-191.

[7] Schurman JV, Friesen CA, Danda CE, Andre L, Welchert E, Lavenbarg T, Cocjin JT, Hyman PE. Diagnosing functional abdominal pain with Rome II criteria: Parent, child, and clinician agreement. J Pediatr Gastroenterol Nutr 2005; 41: 291-295.

[8] Chogle A, Dhroove G, Sztainberg M, Di Lorenzo C, Saps M. How reliable are the Rome III criteria for the assessment of functional gastrointestinal disorders in children? Am J Gastroenterol 2010; 105: 2697-2701.

[9] Schurman JV, Hunter HL, Friesen CA. Conceptualization and treatment of chronic abdominal pain in pediatric gastroenterology practice. J Pediatr Gastroenterol Nutr 2010; 50: 32-37.

[10] Hyams JS, Davis P, Sylvester FA, Zeiter DK, Justinich CJ, Lerer T. Dyspepsia in children and adolescents: A prospective study. J Pediatr Gastroenterol Nutr 2000; 30: 413-418.

[11] Piacentino D, Cantarini R, Alfonsi M, Badiali D, Pallotta N, Biondi M, Corazziari ES. Psychopathological features of irritable bowel syndrome patients with and without functional dyspepsia: A cross sectional study. BMC Gastroenterology 2011; 11: 94.

[12] Schurman JV, Danda CE, Friesen CA, Hyman PE, Simon SD, Cocjin JT. Variations in psychological profile among children with recurrent abdominal pain. J Clin Psych Med Setting 2008; 15: 241-251.

[13] Rippel SW, Acra S, Correa H, Vaezi M, Di Lorenzo C, Walker LS. Pediatric patients with dyspepsia have chronic symptoms, anxiety, and lower quality of life as adolescents and adults. Gastroenterology 2012; 142: 754-761.

[14] Aro P, Talley NJ, Agréus L, Johansson S-E, Bolling-Sternevald E, Storskrubb T, Ronkainen J. Functional dyspepsia impairs quality of life in the adult population. Aliment Pharmacol Ther 2011; 33: 1215-1224.

[15] Mayer EA, Tillisch K. The brain-gut axis in abdominal pain syndromes. Annu Rev Med 2011; 62: 381-396.

[16] Christianson JA, Bielefeldt K, Altier C, Cenac N, Davis BM, Gebhart GF, High KW, Kollarik M, Randich A, Undem B, Vergnolle N. Development, plasticity and modulation of visceral afferents. Brain Res Rev 2009; 60: 171-186.

[17] Al-Chaer ED, Kawasaki M, Pasricha PJ. A new model of chronic visceral hypersensitivity in adult rats induced by colon irritation during postnatal development. Gastroenterology 2000; 119: 1276-1285.

[18] Winston J, Shenoy M, Medley D, Naniwadekar A, Parischka PJ. The vanilloid receptor initiates and maintains colonic hypersensitivity induced by neonatal colon irritation in rats. Gastroenterology 2007; 132: 615-627.

[19] Kokkonen J, Ruuska T, Karttunen TJ, Niinimäki A. mucosal pathology of the forgut associated with food allergy and recurrent abdominal pains in children. Acta Paediatr 2001; 90: 16-21.

[20] Ashorn M, Ruuska T, Karikoski R. Välipakka J, Mäki M. Gastric mucosal cell densities in Helicobacter pylori-positive and –negative dyspeptic children and healthy controls. J Pediatr Gastroenterol Nutr 1994; 18: 146-151.

[21] Canan O, Ozcay F, Ozbay-Hosnut F, Yazici C, Bilezikci B. Value of the Likert dyspepsia scale in differentiation of functional and organic dyspepsia in children. J Pediatr Gastroenterol Nutr. 2011; 52: 392-398.

[22] Friesen CA, Lin Z, Garola R, Andre L, Burchell N, Moore A, Roberts C, McCallum RW. Chronic gastritis is not associated with gastric dysrhythmia or delayed solid emptying in children with dyspepsia. Dig Dis Sci 2005; 50: 1012-1018.

[23] Hall W, Buckley M, Crotty P, O'Morain CA. Gastric mucosal mast cells are increased in Helicobacter pylori-negative functional dyspepsia. Clin Gastroenterol Hepatol 2003; 1: 363-369.

[24] Choi MG, Park SJ, Lee SY, Cho YK, Park JM, Han HW, Oh JW, Lee IS, Chung IS. Association of psychological factors with activation of mucosal immune system in functional dyspepsia. Neurogastroenterol Motil 2004; 16: 668.

[25] Nakajima H, Krishnan B, Ota H, Segura AM, Hattori A, Graham DY, Genta RM. Mast cell involvement in gastritis with or without Helicobacter pylori infection. Gastroenterology 1997; 113: 746-754.

[26] Walker MM, Talley NJ, Prabhakar M, Pennaneac'h CJ, Aro P, Ronkainen J, Storskrubb T, Harmsen WS, Zinmeister AR, Agreus L. Duodenal mastocytosis, eosinophilia and intraepithelial lymphocytosis as possible disease markers in the irritable bowel syndrome and functional dyspepsia. Aliment Pharmacol Ther 2009; 29: 765-773.

[27] Hou X-H, Zhu L-R, Li Q-X, Chen JDZ. Alterations in mast cells and 5-HT positive cells in gastric mucosa in functional dyspepsia patients with hypersensitivity. Neurogastroenterol Motil 2001; 13: 398-399.

[28] Friesen CA, Lin Z, Singh M, Singh V, Schurman JV, Burchell N, Cocjin JT, McCallum RW. Antral inflammatory cells, gastric emptying, and electrogastrography in pediatric functional dyspepsia. Dig Dis Sci 2008; 53: 2634-2640.

[29] Friesen CA, Lin Z, Hyman PE, Andre L, Welchert E, Schurman JV, Cocjin JT, Burchell N, Pulliam S, Moore A, Lavenbarg T, McCallum RW. Electrogastrography in pediatric functional dyspepsia: Relationship to gastric emptying and symptom severity. J Pediatr Gastroenterol Nutr 2006; 42: 265-269.

[30] Lowichik A, Weinberg AG. A quantitative evaluation of mucosal eosinophils in the pediatric gastrointestinal tract. Modern Pathology 1996; 9: 110-114.

[31] Kalach N, Huvenne H, Gosset P, Papadopopoulos S, Dehecq E, Decoster A, Creusy C, Dupont C. Eosinophil counts in the upper digestive mucosa of Western European children: variations with age, organs, symptoms, Helicobacter pylori status, and pathologic findings. J Pediatr Gastroenterol Nutr 2011; 52: 175-182.

[32] Erjefalt JS, Greiff L, Andersson M, Adelroth E, Jeffrey PK, Persson CGA. Degranulation pattern of eosinophil granulocytes as determinants of eosinophil driven disease. Thorax 2001; 56: 341-344.

[33] Friesen CA, Andre L, Garola R, Hodge C, Roberts C. Activated duodenal mucosal eosinophils in children with dyspepsia: A pilot transmission electron microscopic study. J Pediatr Gastroenterol Nutr 2002; 35: 329-333.

[34] Talley NJ, Walker MM, Aro P, Ronkainen J, Storskrubb T, Hindley LA, Harmsen WS, Zinsmeister AR, Agréus L. Non-ulcer dyspepsia and duodenal eosinophilia: An adult endoscopic population-based case-control study. Clin Gastroenterol Hepatol 2007; 5: 1175-1183.

[35] Walker MM, Talley NJ, Prabhakar M, Pennaneac'h CJ, Aro P, Ronkainen J, Storskrubb T, Harmsen WS, Zinsmeister AR, Agreus L. Duodenal mastocytosis, eosinophilia and intraepithelial lymphocytosis as possible disease markers in the irritable

bowel syndrome and functional dyspepsia. Aliment Pharmacol Ther 2009; 29: 765-773.

[36] Walker MM, Salehian SS, Murray CE, Rajendran A, Hoare JM, Negus R, Powell N, Talley NJ. Implications of eosinophilia in the normal duodenal biopsy: An association with allergy and functional dyspepsia. Aliment Pharmacol Ther 2010; 31: 1229-1236.

[37] Thakkar K, Chen L, Tatevian N, Schulman RJ, McDuffie A, Tsou M, Gilger MA, El-Serag HB. Diagnostic yield of oesophagogastroduodenoscopy in children with abdominal pain. Aliment Pharmacol Ther 2009; 30: 662-669.

[38] Friesen CA, Neilan NA, Schurman JV, Taylor DL, Kearns GL, Abdel-Rahman SM. Montelukast in the treatment of duodenal eosinophilia in children with dyspepsia: Effect on eosniophil density and activation in relation to pharmacokinetics. BMC Gastroenterol 2009; 9: 32.

[39] Liu L, Li Q, Sapolsky R, Liao M, Mehta K, Bhargava A, Pasricha P. Transient gastric irritation in the neonatal rats leads to changes in hypothalamic CRF expression, depression- and anxiety-like behavior as adults. PLoS One 2011; 6: e19498.

[40] Chrousos GP. Stress, chronic inflammation, and emotional and physical well-being: concurrent effects and chronic sequelae. J All Clin Immunol 2000; 106: S275-S291.

[41] Fukudo S, Nomura T, Hongo M. Impact of corticotrophin-releasing hormone on gastrointestinal motility and adrenocorticotropic hormone in normal controls and patients with irritable bowel syndrome. Gut 1999; 42: 845-849.

[42] Dickhaus B, Mayer EA, Firooz, Stains J, Conde F, Olivas TI, Fass R, Chang L, Mayer M, Naliboff BD. Irritable bowel syndrome patients show enhanced modulation of visceral perception by auditory stress. Am J Gastroenterol 2003; 98: 135-143.

[43] Posserud I, Agerforz P, Ekman R, Bjornsson ES, Abrahamsson H, Simren M. Altered visceral perceptual and neuroendocrine response in patients with irritable bowel syndrome during mental stress. Gut 2004; 53: 1102-1108.

[44] Bohmelt AH, Nater UM, Franke S, Hellhammer DH, Ehlert U. Basal and stimulated hypothalamic-pituitary-adrenal axis activity in patients with functional gastrointestinal disorders and healthy controls. Psychosom Med 2005; 67: 288-294.

[45] Dinan TG, Quigley EMM, Ahmed SMM, Scully P, O'Brien S, O'Mahony L, O'Mahony S, Shanahan F, Keeling PWN. Hypothalamic-pituitary-gut axis dysregulation in irritable bowel syndrome: plasma cytokines as a potential biomarker? Gastroenterology 2006; 130: 304-311.

[46] Wallon C, Söderholm JD. Corticotropin-releasing hormone and mast cells in the regulation of mucosal barrier function in the human colon. Ann N Y Acad Sci 2009; 1165: 206-210.

[47] Zheng P-Y, Feng B-S, Oluwole C, Struiksma S, Chen X, Li P, Tang S-G, Yang P-C. Psychological stress induces eosinophils to produce corticotrophin releasing hormone in the intestine. Gut 2009; 58: 1473-1479.

[48] Friesen CA, Schurman JV, Qadeer A, Andre L, Welchert E, Cocjin J. Relationship between mucosal eosinophils and anxiety in pediatric dyspepsia. Gastroenterology 2005; 129: A-158.

[49] Walker MM, Warwick A, Ung C, Talley NJ. The role of eosinophils and mast cells in intestinal functional disease. Curr Gastroenterol Rep 2011; 13: 323-330.

[50] He S-H. Key role of mast cells and their major secretory products in inflammatory bowel disease. World J Gastroenterol 2004; 10: 309-318.

[51] Hall W, Buckley M, Crotty P, O'Morain CA. Gastric mucosal mast cells are increased in Helicobacter pylori-negative functional dyspepsia. Clin Gastroenterol Hepatol 2003; 1: 363-369.

[52] Santos J, Saperas E, Nogueiras C, Mourelle M, Antolin M, Cadahia A, Malagelada J-R. Release of mast cell mediators into the jejunum by cold pain stress in humans. Gastroenterology 1998; 114: 640-648.

[53] Coruzzi G, Adami M, Pozzoli C. Role of histamine H4 receptors in the gastrointestinal tract. Frontiers Biosci 2012; S4: 226-239.

[54] Van Oudenhove L, Tack J. New epidemiologic evidence on functional dyspepsia subgroups and their relationship to psychosocial dysfunction. Gastroenterology 2009; 137: 23-26.

[55] Zanini B, Ricci C, Bandera F, Caselani F, Magni A, Laronga AM, Lanzini A. Incidence of post-infectious irritable bowel syndrome and functional intestinal disorders following a water-borne viral gastroenteritis outbreak. Am J Gastroenterol 2012; 107: 891-899.

[56] Ford AC, Thabane M, Collins SM, Moayyedi P, Garg AX, Clark WF, Marshall JK. Prevalence of uninvestigated dyspepsia 8 years after a large waterborne outbreak of bacterial dysentery: A cohort study. Gastroenterology 2010; 138: 1727-1736.

[57] Hanevik K, Dizdar V, Langeland N, Hausken T. Development of functional gastrointestinal disorders after Giardia lamblia infection. BMC Gastroenterol 2009; 9: 27.

[58] Saps M, Pensabene L, Di Martino L, Staiano A, Wechsler J, Zheng X, Di Lorenzo C. Post-infectious functional gastrointestinal disorders in children. J Pediatr 2008; 152: 812-816.

[59] Sarnelli G, Vandenberghe J, Tack J. Visceral hypersensitivity in functional disorders of the upper gastrointestinal tract. Dig Liv Dis 2004; 36: 371-376.

[60] Suzuki H. Post-infectious functional dyspepsia- A novel disease entity among functional gastrointestinal disorders- relation to Helicobacter pylori infection? Neurogastroenterol Motil 2009; 21: 832-e56.

[61] Mearin F. Postinfectious functional gastrointestinal disorders. J Clin Gastroenterol 2011; 45: S102-S105.

[62] Futagami S, Shindo T, Kawagoe T, Horie A, Shimpuku M, Gudis K, Iwakiri K, Itoh T, Sakamoto C. Migration of eosinophils and CCR2/CD68-double positive cells into duodenal mucosa of patients with postinfectious functional dyspepsia. Am J Gastroenterol 2010; 105: 1835-1842.

[63] Kindt S, Tertychnyy A, de Hertogh G, Geboes K, Tack J. Intestinal immune activation in presumed post-infectious functional dyspepsia. Neurogastroenterol Motil 2009; 21: 832-e56.

[64] Li X, Chen H, Lu H, Li W, Chen X, Peng Y, Ge Z. The study of the role of inflammatory cells and mediators in post-infectious functional dyspepsia. Scand J Gastroenterol 2010; 45: 573-581.

[65] Jin X, Li YM. Systematic review and meta-analysis from Chinese literature: the association between Helicobacter pylori eradication and improvement of functional dyspepsia. Helicobacter 2007; 12: 541-546.

[66] Gwee KA, Teng L, Wong RK, Ho KY, Sutedja DS, Yeoh KG. The response of Asian patients with functional dyspepsia to eradication of Helicobacter pylori infection. Eur J Gastroenterol Hepatol 2009, 21: 417-424.

[67] Lan L, Yu J, Chen Y-L, Zhong Y-L, Zhang H, Jia C-H, Yuan Y, Liu B-W. Symptom-based tendencies of Helicobacter pylori eradication in patients with functional dyspepsia. World J Gastroenterol 2011; 17: 3242-3247.

[68] Mazzoleni LE, Sander GB, de Magalháes Francesconi CF, Mazzoleni F, Uchoa DM, De Bona LR, Milbradt TC, Von Reisswitz PS, Berwanger O, Bressel M, Edelweiss MI, Marini SS, Molina CG, Folador L, Lunkes RP, Heck R, Birkhan OA, Spindler BM, Katz N, da Silveira Colombo B, Guerrieri PP, Renck LB, Grando E, de Moura BH, Dahmer FD, Rauber J, Prolla JC. Helicobacter pylori eradication in functional dyspepsia. HEROES trial. Arch Intern Med 2011; 171: 1929-1936.

[69] Moayyedi P, Soo S, Deeks J, Delaney B, Harris A, Innes M, Oakes R, Wilson S, Roalfe A, Bennerr C, Forman D. Eradication of Helicobacter pylori for non-ulcer dyspepsia. Cochrane Database Syst Rev 2006, CD002096.

[70] Sugano K. Should we still subcategorize Helicobacter pylori-associated dyspepsia as functional disease? J Neurogastroenterol Motil 2011; 17: 366-371.

[71] Mirbagheri SA, Khajavirad N, Rakhshani N, Ostovaneh MR, Hoseini SME, Hoseini V. Impact of Helicobacter pylori infection and microscopic duodenal histopathologi-

cal changes on clinical symptoms of patients with functional dyspepsia. Dig Dis Sci 2012; 57: 967-972.

[72] Turkkan E, Uslan I, Acarturk G, Topak N, Kahraman A, Dilek FH, Akcan Y, Karaman O, Colbay M, Yuksel S. Does Helicobacter pylori-induced inflammation of gastric mucosa determine the severity of symptoms in functional dyspepsia? J Gastroenterol 2009; 44: 66-70.

[73] Hofman V, Lassalle S, Selva E, Kalem K, Steff A, Hébuterne X, Sicard D, Auberger P, Hofman P. Involvement of mast cells in gastritis caused by Helicobacter pylori: a potential role in epithelial cell apoptosis. J Clin Pathol 2007; 60: 600-607.

[74] Moorchung N, Srivastava AN, Gupta NK, Malaviya AK, Achyut BR, Mittal B. The role of mast cells and eosinophils in chronic gastritis. Clin Exp Med 2006; 6: 107-114.

[75] Aydemir S, Tekin IO, Numanoglu G, Borazan A, Ustundag Y. Eosinophil infiltration, gastric juice and serum eosinophil cationic protein levels in Helicobacter pylori-associated chronic gastritis and gastric ulcer. Mediators of Inflammation 2004; 13: 369-372.

[76] Kalach N, Huvenne H, Gosset P, Papadopoulos S, Dehecq E, Decoster A, Creusy C, Dupont C. Eosinophil counts in upper digestive mucosa of Western European children: Variation with age, organs, symptoms, Helicobacter pylori status, and pathological findings. J Pediatr Gastroenterol Nutr. 2011; 52: 175-182.

[77] Azpiroz F, Bouin M, Camilleri M, Mayer EA, Poitras P, Serra J, Spiller RC. Mechanisms of hypersensitivity in IBS and functional disorders. Neurogastroenterol Motil 2007; 19 (Supl 1):62-68.

[78] Ang TL, Fock KM, Teo EK, Chan YH, Ng TM, Chua TS, Tan JY. Helicobacter pylori eradication versus prokinetics in the treatment of functional dyspepsia: a randomized, double-blind study. J Gastroenterol 2006; 41: 647-653.

[79] Lin Z, Chen JDZ, Parolisi S, Shifflett J, Peura DA, McCallum RW. Prevalence of gastric myoelectrical abnormalities in patients with nonulcer dyspepsia and H. pylori infection. Resolution after H. pylori eradication. Dig Dis Sci 2001; 46: 739-745.

[80] Saps M, Lu P, Bonilla S. Cow's-milk allergy is a risk factor for the development of FGIDs in children. J Pediatr Gastroenterol Nutr 2011; 52: 166-169.

[81] Schäppi MG, Borrelli O, Knafelz D, Williams S, Smithy VV, Milla PJ, Lindley KJ. Mast cell-nerve interactions in children with functional dyspepsia. J Pediatr Gastroenterol Nutr 2008; 47: 472-480.

[82] Murch S. Allergy and intestinal dysmotility: evidence of genuine causal linkage? Curr Opin Gastroenterol 2006; 22: 664-668.

[83] Mansueto P, Iacono G, Seidita A, D'Alcamo A, Sprini D, Carroccio A. Review article: intestinal lymphoid nodular hyperplasia in children- the relationship to food hypersensitivity. Aliment Pharmacol Ther 2012; 35: 1000-1009.

[84] Ravelli AM, Tobanelli P, Volpi S, Ugazio AG. Vomiting and gastric motility in infants with cow's milk allergy. J Pediatr Gastroenterol Nutr 2001; 32: 59-64.

[85] Neilan N, Dowling PJ, Taylor DL, Ryan P, Schurman JV, Friesen CA. Useful biomarkers in pediatric eosinophilic duodenitis. Do they exist? J Pediatr Gastroenterol Nutr 2010; 50: 377-384.

[86] Magnusson J, Lin XP, Dahlman-Höglund A, Hanson LÅ, Telemo E, Magnusson O, Bengtsson U, Ahlstedt S. Seasonal intestinal inflammation in patients with birch pollen allergy. J Allergy Clin Immunol 2003; 112: 45-51.

[87] Edsbäcker S, Andersson T. Pharmacokinetics of budesonide (Entocort EC) capsules for Crohn's disease. Clin Pharmacokinet 2004; 43: 803-821.

[88] Siewert E, Lammert F, Koppitz P, Schmidt T, Matern S. Eosinophilic gastroenteritis with severe protein-losing enteropathy: successful treatment with budesonide. Dig Liver Dis 2006; 38: 55-59.

[89] Elsing C, Placke J, Gross-Weege W. Budesonide for the treatment of obstructive eosinophilic jejunitis. Z Gastroenterol 2007; 45: 187-189.

[90] Shahzad G, Moise D, Lipka S, Rizvon K, Mustacchia PJ. Eosinophilic enterocolitis diagnosed by means of upper endoscoy and colonoscopy with random biopsies treated with budesonide: A case report and review of the literature. ISRN Gastroenterology 2011; doi:10.5402/2011/608901

[91] Friesen CA, Sandridge L, Andre L, Roberts CC, Abdel-Rahman SM. Mucosal eosinophilia and response to H1/H2 antagonist and cromolyn therapy in pediatric dyspepsia. Clin Pediatr 2006; 45: 143-147.

[92] Lunardi C, Bambara LM, Biasi D, Cortina P, Peroli P, Nicolis F, Favari F, Pacor ML. Double-blind cross-over trial of oral sodium cromoglycate in patients with irritable bowel syndrome due to food intolerance. Clin Exp Allergy 1991; 21: 569-572.

[93] Stefanini GF, Prati E, Albini MC, Piccinini G, Capelli S, Castelli E, Mazzetti M, Gasbarrini G. Oral disodium cromoglycate treatment on irritable bowel syndrome: An open study on 101 subjects with diarrheic type. Am J Gastroenterol 1992; 87: 55-57.

[94] Stefanini GF, Saggioro A, Alvisi V, Angelini G, Capurso L, di Lorenzo G, Dobrilla G, Dodero M, Galimberti M, Gasbaffini G, Manghisi O, Marsigli L, Mazzaca G, Rigo L, Sacerdoti G, Scolozzi R, Surrenti C, Grazioli I, Melzi G. Oral cromolyn sodium in comparison to elimination diet in the irritable bowel syndrome, diarrheic type. Multicenter study of 428 patients. Scand J Gastroenterol 1995, 30: 535-541.

[95] Klooker TK, Braak B, Koopman KE, Welting O, Wouters MM, van der Heide S, Schemann M, Bischoff SC, van den Wijngaard RM, Boeckxstaens GE. The mast cell stabil-

izer ketotifen decreases visceral hypersensitivity and improves intestinal symptoms in patients with irritable bowel syndrome. Gut 2010; 59: 1213-1221.

[96] See MC, Birnbaum AH, Schechter CB, Goldenberg MM, Benkov KJ. Double-blind, placebo-controlled trial of famotidine in children with abdominal pain and dyspepsia. Dig Dis Sci 2001; 46: 985-992.

[97] Dehghani SM, Imanieh MH, Oboodi R, Haghighat M. The comparative study of the effectiveness of cimetidine, ranitidine, famotidine, and omeperazole in treatment of children with dyspepsia. ISRN Pediatrics 2011; doi:10.5402/2011/219287.

[98] Kato M, Watanabe M, Konishi S, Kudo M, Konno J, Meguro T, Kitamori S, Nakagawa S, Shimizu Y, Takeda H, Asaka M. Randomized, double-blind, placebo-controlled crossover trial of famotidine in patients with functional dyspepsia. Aliment Pharmacol Ther 2005; 21 (Suppl. 2): 27-31.

[99] Amini M, Chehreh MEG, Khedmat H, Valizadegan G, Babaei M, Darvishi A, Taheri S. Famotidine in the treatment of functional dyspepsia: A randomized double-blind, placebo-controlled trial. J Egypt Pub Health Assoc 2012; 87: 29-33.

[100] Seno H, Nakase H, Chiba T. Usefulness of famotidine in functional dyspepsia patient treatment: comparison among prokinetic, acid suppression and antianxiety therapies. Aliment Pharmacol Ther 2005; 21 (Suppl 2): 32-36.

[101] Veldhuyzen van Zanten SJO, Chiba N, Armstrong D, Barkun A, Thomson A, Smyth S, Escobedo S, Lee J, Sinclair P. A randomized trial comparing omeperazole, ranitidine, cisapride, or placebo in Helicobacter pylori negative, primary cate patients with dyspepsia: The CADET-HN study. Am J Gastroenterol 2005; 100: 1477-1488.

[102] Wang WH, Huang JQ, Zheng GEF, Xia HHX, Wong WM, Liu XG, Karlberg J, Wong BCY. Effects of proton-pump inhibitors on functional dyspepsia: A meta-analysis of randomized placebo-controlled trials. Clin Gastroenterol Hepatol 2007; 5: 178-185.

[103] Talley NJ, Meineche-Schmidt V, Paré P, Duckworth M, Räisänen P, Pap A, Kordecki H, Schmid V. Efficacy of omeperazole in functional dyspepsia: double-blind, randomized, placebo-controlled trials (the Bond and Opera studies). Aliment Pharmacol Ther 1998; 12: 1055-1065.

[104] Peura DA, Kovacs TOG, Metz DC, Siepman N, Pilmer BL, Talley NJ. Lansoprazole in the treatment of functional dyspepsia: Two double-blind, randomized, placebo-controlled trials. Am J Med 2004; 116: 740-748.

[105] Van Rensburg C, Berghöfer P, Enns R, Dattani ID, Martiz JF, Carro PG, Fischer R, Schwan T. Efficacy and safety of pantoprazole 20 mg once daily treatment in patients with ulcer-like functional dyspepsia. Curr Med Res Opin 2008; 24: 2009-2018.

[106] Kamiya T, Shikano M, Tanaka M, Tsukamoto H, Ebi M, Hirata Y, Mizushima T, Murakami K, Shimura T, Mizoshita T, Mori Y, Tanida S, Kato T, Imaeda K, Kataoka H,

Joh T. The effect of omeperazole on gastric myoelectrical activity and emptying. J Smooth Musc Res 2011; 47: 79-87.

[107] Milenov K, Todorov S, Vassileva M, Zamfirova R, Shahbazian A. Interaction between histaminergic and cholinergic pathways of gastric motility regulation. Methods Find Exp Clin Pharmacol 1996; 18: 33-39.

[108] Izzo AA, Costa M, Mascolo N, Capasso F. The role of histamine H1, H2, and H3 receptors on enteric ascending synaptic transmission in the guinea pig ileum. J Pharmacol Exp Ther 1998; 287: 952-957.

[109] Jiang W, Kreis ME, Eastwood C, Kirkup AJ, Humphrey PP, Grundy D. 5-HT(3) and histamine H(1) receptors mediate afferent nerve sensitivity to intestinal anaphylaxis in rats. Gastroenterology 2000; 119: 1267-1275.

[110] Moharana AK, Bhattacharya SK, Mediratta PK, Sharma KK. Possible role of histamine receptors in the central regulation of immune responses. Indian J Physiol Pharmacol 2000; 44: 153-160.

[111] Wood JD. Neuropathophysiology of irritable bowel syndrome. J Clin Gastroenterol 2002; 35 (Suppl): 11-22.

[112] Matter SE, Bhatia PS, Miner PB. Evaluation of antral mast cell in nonulcer dyspepsia. Dig Dis Sci 1990; 35: 1358-1363.

[113] Lllorca PM, Spadone C, Sol O, Danniau A, Bougerol T, Corruble E, Faruch M, Macher JP, Sermet E, Servant D. Efficacy and safety of hydroxyzine in the treatment of generalized anxiety disorder: A 3-month double-blind study. J Clin Psychiatry 2002; 63:1020-1027.

[114] Holgate ST, Sampson AP. Antileukotriene therapy: Future directions. Am J Respir Crit Care Med 2000; 161: S147-S153Mellor EA, Austen KF, Boyce JA. Cysteinyl leukotrienes and uridine diphosphate induce cytokine generation by human mast cells through an interleukin 4-regulated pathway that is inhibited by leukotriene receptor antagonists. J Exp Med 2002; 195: 583-592.

[115] Mellor EA, Austen KF, Boyce JA. Cysteinyl leukotrienes and uridine diphosphate induce cytokine generation by human mast cells through an interleukin 4-regulated pathway that is inhibited by leukotriene receptor antagonists. J Exp Med 2002; 195: 583-592.

[116] Goldenberg MM, Subers EM. The effect of leukotriene D4 on the isolated stomach and colon of the rat. Life Sci 1983; 33: 2121-2127.

[117] Burakoff R, Nastos E, Won S, Percy WH. Comparison of the effects of leukotrienes B4 and D4 on distal colonic motility in the rabbit in vivo. Am J Physiol 1989; 257 (6 Pt 1): G860-G864.

[118] Freedman SM, Wallace JL, Shaffer EA. Characterization of leukotriene-induced contraction of the guinea-pig gallbladder in vitro. Can J Physiol Pharmacol 1993; 71: 145-150.

[119] Goldhill JM, Finkelman FD, Morris SC, Shea-Donohue T. Neural control of mouse small intestinal longitudinal muscle: Interactions with inflammatory mediators. J Pharmacol Exp Ther 1995; 274: 72-77.

[120] Frieling T, Becker K, Rupprecht C, Dobreva G, Häussinger D, Schemann M. Leukotriene-evoked cyclic chloride secretion is mediated by enteric neuronal modulation in guinea-pig colon. Naunyn Schmiedebergs Arch Pharmacol 1997; 355: 625-630.

[121] Kim N, Cao W, Song IS, Dim C, Sohn UD, Harnett KM, Biancani P. Leukotriene D4-induced contraction of cat esophageal and lower esophageal sphincter circular smooth muscle. Gastroenterology 1998; 115: 919-928.

[122] Liu S, Hu HZ, Gao C, Gao N, Wang G, Wang X, Gao X, Xia Y, Wood JD. Actions of cysteinyl leukotrienes in the enteric nervous system of guinea-pig stomach and small intestine. Eur J Pharmacol 2003; 459: 27-39.

[123] Liu S, Hu H-Z, Gao N, Gao C, Wang G, Wang X, Peck OC, Kim G, Gao X, Xia Y, Wood JD. Neuroimmune interactions in guinea pig stomach and small intestine. Am J Physiol Gastrointest Liver Physiol 2003; 284: G154-G164.

[124] Friesen CA, Kearns GL, Andre L, Neustrom M, Roberts CC, Abdel-Rahman SM. Clinical efficacy and pharmacokinetics of montelukast in dyspeptic children with duodenal eosinophilia. J Pediatr Gastroenterol Nutr 2004; 38: 343-351.

[125] Friesen CA, Neilan NA, Schurman JV, Taylor DL, Kearns GL, Abdel-Rahman SM. Montelukast in the treatment of duodenal eosinophilia in children with dyspepsia: Effect on eosinophil density and activation in relation to pharmacokinetics. BMC Gastroenterol 2009; 9: 32.

[126] Bischoff SC, Lorentz A, Schwengberg S, Weier G, Raab R, Manns MP. Mast cells are an important cellular source of tumor necrosis factor alpha in human intestinal tissue. Gut 1999; 44: 643-652.

[127] Thomas PS, Heywood G. Effects of inhaled tumor necrosis factor alpha in subjects with mild asthma. Thorax 2002; 57: 774-778.

[128] Liu LY, Bates ME, Jarjour NN, Busse WW, Bertics PJ, Kelly EA. Generation of Th1 and Th2 chemokines by human eosinophils: Evidence for a critical role of TNF-alpha. J Immunol 2007; 179: 4840-4848.

[129] Turner D, Wolters VM, Russell RK, Shakhnovich V, Muise AM, Ledder O, Ngan B, Friesen C. Anti-TNF, infliximab and adalimumab, can be effective in eosinophilic bowel disease: A report of eight pediatric cases. J Pediatr Gastroenterol Nutr; doi: 10.1097/MPG.0b013e3182801e60.

[130] Humphreys PA, Gevirtz RN. Treatment of recurrent abdominal pain: Components analysis of four treatment protocols. J Pediatr Gastroenterol Nutr 2000; 31: 47-51.

[131] Schurman JV, Wu YP, Grayson P, Friesen CA. A pilot study to assess the efficacy of biofeedback-assisted relaxation training as an adjunct treatment for pediatric functional dyspepsia associated with duodenal eosinophilia. J Pediatr Psychol 2010; 35: 837-847.

Chapter 4

Functional Dyspepsia and *Helicobacter pylori* Infection

Ratha-korn Vilaichone and Varocha Mahachai

Additional information is available at the end of the chapter

http://dx.doi.org/10.5772/56652

1. Introduction

Helicobacter pylori (*H. pylori*) was first observed over 100 years ago yet its association with clinical diseases was not fully understanding until 1982 when Marshall and Warren identified and subsequently cultured the gastric bacterium. At their first attempt to culture the bacteria was not successful. Colonies finally grew when they accidentally left some culture plates over the Easter holiday. Dr. Barry Marshall subsequently inoculated himself with culture broth containing more than 1 billion organism to prove that this bacterium would cause peptic ulcers supporting Koch's postulate. He developed acute gastritis 1 week after the inoculation. *H. pylori* is a microaerophilic, spiral shaped, gram negative bacterium measuring about 3.5 microns in length and 0.5 microns in width. In vitro, this bacterium is a gradually growing organism that can be cultured on blood agar incubated at 37ºC in a microaerophilic condition (5% oxygen) for 4-7 days. The colony of this bacteria is tiny, uniformly sized and translucence (fig 2A).

H. pylori is a Gram-negative, spiral shaped, bacterium about 3.5 microns long and 0.5 microns wide. (fig 2B). This bacterium uses its 2-7 unipolar flagella to escape the harsh luminal acidity by burrowing into the mucus layer that covers the gastric mucosa and so reside in close proximity to the more neutral pH of the epithelial cell surface of the gastric mucosa. It can convert from a highly motile, helical (spiral) shape to a more dormant coccoidal form, perhaps a survival benefit depending upon its local environment. Being microaerophilic, *H. pylori* requires oxygen. *H. pylori* is biochemically characterized as positive for catalase, oxidase, and urease. The urease enzyme, which has been located on the surface of the bacteria, is important and likely to be vital for bacterial survival and colonization in the highly acidity milieu of the stomach. Urease breaks down the luminal urea normally produced by the gastric mucosa, yielding carbon dioxide and ammonia.

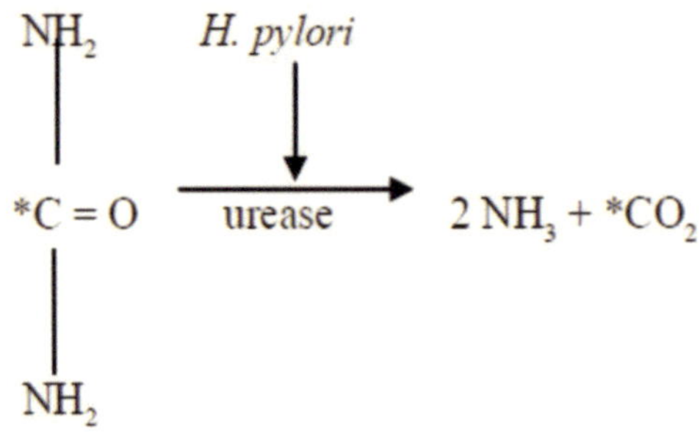

Figure 1. or 14C-urea is hydrolyzed by the *H pylori* urease enzyme and can be detected by CO2 in breath samples

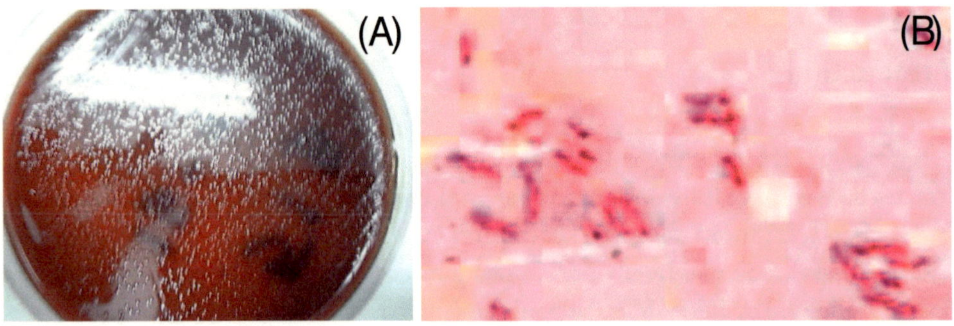

Figure 2. A) *H. pylori* colonies; (B). *H. pylori* detected by gram stain

Ammonia then accepts a proton (H^+), lessening the nearby acidity and forming protective surroundings that allow its survival. Furthermore, urease activity is clinically relevance in the form of several tests to diagnose infection such as rapid urease test and urea breath test. [1-4] The ammonia produced however is toxic to the epithelium, and aided by other products like proteases, vacuolating cytotoxin A (associated with cytotoxin-associated gene A), and certain phospholipases damages the mucosa. *H. pylori* infection also increases gastric acid secretion (suppressing somatostatin to allow increased gastrin), down regulates mucosal defense mechanisms and elicits an inflammatory response.

H. pylori infects the gastric mucosa in 20-80 % of humans throughout the world, making it a very common bacterial infection. In developing countries, the infection tends to be acquired via the fecal-oral or oral-oral route during childhood and subsequently persists through adulthood. In developed countries, childhood infection is no longer common (rare under 10 years of age) though prevalence does increase during adulthood (>50% if over 50 years); the latter cohort likely acquired H. pylori during childhood. This bacteria is the major pathologic agent in the development of gastritis, gastric ulcer, duodenal ulcer, MALT lymphoma and gastric cancer. The International Agency for Research into Cancer has classified *H. pylori* as a class 1 carcinogen which is in the same class as cigarette smoke. [1-3]

Functional dyspepsia (FD) is one of the most common causes of dyspeptic symptoms. FD is recognized as heterogeneous group of symptoms located in the center of upper abdomen. The prevalence of dyspepsia is variable in different populations and environmental factors. In 2006 the Rome III provides the diagnostic criteria, which are included one or more of the following [5, 6]

1. Bothersome postprandial fullness
2. Early satiation
3. Epigastric pain
4. Epigastric burning

The FD patient must not have any evidence of structural disease to explain the dyspeptic symptoms. Symptom onset should occur at least 6 months prior to diagnosis while the criteria must be fulfilled for the last 3 months. FD also can be divided into two major syndromes: the postprandial distress syndrome and the epigastric pain syndrome. The postprandial distress syndrome type of FD constitutes bothersome postprandial fullness and early satiation, occurring after meal and at least several times per week. Upper abdominal bloating or postprandial nausea or excessive belching might be present. In contrast, the epigastric pain syndrome type of FD mostly suffers with intermittent epigastric pain or burning at least once a week. The pain should not refer to other abdominal or chest regions, and should not be relieved by defecation of passage of flatus. [5]

2. Epidemiology of *H. pylori* infection and FD

H. pylori is a global bacterial infection. Its prevalence varies greatly from 10-80% between countries, being quite elevated in developing countries in Asia, Africa, and South America but rather low in North America and Western Europe. In developed countries, approximately 20% of the population under the age of 40 years and 50% of those over the age of 60 years carry the infection. [6]

The prevalence of *H. pylori* infection also varies depending on age, socioeconomic status, sanitation and ethnic group [4, 7-9]. Typically, the infection is acquired in childhood before the age of 10 and the rate of acquisition is related inversely to household hygiene and the general levels of sanitation; wherever sanitation and standards of living have improved, the incidence of transmission has declined. The low prevalence in middle and upper socioeconomic populations in Western Europe and North America reflect better sanitation and quality of living. In the United States, the prevalence rate is approximately 50% in African Americans, 60% in Mexican Americans, and 26% in whites. [4] In developing countries, the prevalence among adult people is between 50-80%.

H. pylori infection may be evident in 20-60% of patients with functional dyspepsia, but the clinical relevance in most instances is confounded by the background frequency of this bacteria in the general population. A large scale nationwide community-based endoscopic survey of 2,488 adult subjects identified an overall *H. pylori* infection at 40.2% that was no different in dyspeptic subjects compared to asymptomatic persons. Differences amongst geographic regions likely related to differences in socioeconomic status and community hygiene during childhood period. [8] The frequency of functional dyspepsia is common in Asia, varying between 8-23% in most reported studies. [10] In fact, given the common frequency of *H. pylori* infection and challenges in obtaining endoscopy to eliminate organic causes of dyspepsia, it is difficult to discern the extent this microorganism is the basis for dyspepsia in Asia. [10, 11]

There are many FD patients in Asian as well as Western countries. The reported prevalence of *H. pylori* infection in patients with FD varies from 39% to 87%. [14] Several epidemiological studies have shown that *H. pylori* infection occurs more frequently in FD than in matched control populations. A meta-analysis published in 1999 reported a summary odds ratio for *H. pylori* infection in FD of 1.6 (95% CI, 1.4 to 1.8). [15]

3. Pathogenesis of functional dyspepsia associated with *H. pylori* infection

The pathophysiological disturbances generally responsible for the dyspepsia focus on hyperacidity, impaired gastric accommodation (the "stiff fundus") and delayed gastric emptying. FD patients who are infected with *H. pylori* have higher stimulated gastric acid secretion than *H. pylori*-negative healthy volunteers. [16] Impaired accommodation to a meal may be common in functional dyspepsia and early satiety, but is not particularly associated with *H. pylori* positivity or delayed gastric emptying. There is no constituent disturbance of sensory or motor function yet reported in H. pylori-infected persons. Another factor possibly responsible for the dyspepsia associated with H. pylori infection is the gut hormone, ghrelin. Secreted from oxyntic cells, ghrelin normally stimulates gastric motility and food intake. Patients with *H. pylori* may have reduction in ghrelin secretion that might lead to impaired gastric emptying and symptoms of postprandial dyspepsia.

Recent study demonstrated that metronidazole resistant strains of *H. pylori* infection were significantly higher in PDS than those of EPS patients. This study also indicated more specific of *cagA* genotype that presence of *cagA 2a* gene of *H. pylori* infection was significantly higher in metronidazole resistant than those of metronidazole sensitive strains especially in EPS patients. This finding might be helpful to identify metronidazole resistant by using *cagA* genotype in dyspeptic patients. [17]

CagA is a highly immunogenic protein encoded by the *cagA* gene, located at end of the *cag* pathogenicity island (PAI). Infection with *cagA*-positive strains was associated with a greater inflammatory response and an increased risk of adverse clinical outcomes than with *cagA*-negative strains. [7, 18-20] Taneike et al recently reported that the metronidazole resistant rate in *cagA* negative group was significantly higher than in *cagA* positive group and suggested that absence of *cagA* might be a risk factor in development of metronidazole resistance. [21] Unlike many countries such as European countries and United State of America, nearly all of *H. pylori* strains in Thailand possess *cagA*-positive strains. [16] These different results might be explained by variation in *cagA* between the Asian- and Western-types. *CagA* genotype can be divided into *cagA 1a* and *2a* [17] and *cagA 1a* strain of *H. pylori* demonstrated more virulence and associated with more gastric inflammation due to activation of proinflammatory cytokines such as increased production of IL-1β and IL-8 in the gastric mucosa. [21] Previous meta-analysis study reported that *cagA*-positive strain increases the likelihood of successful eradication. [22] The mechanism for the effect of *cagA* on eradication outcome might be explained by the presence of *cagA* induces secretion of inflammatory cytokine in gastric epithelial cells and increased gastric inflammatory response. [22] Consequently, the increase blood flow may help in the diffusion of antibiotics. [23] Another possibility might be explained by the density of *H. pylori* in gastric mucosa which has been reported to be higher in *cagA*-positive strains than *cagA*-negative strains, thus *cagA*-positive strains might be proliferative faster than *cagA*-negative strains. [24, 25] As antibiotics are more active on rapidly growing bacteria, *cagA*-positive strains would be more susceptible to antibiotic activity [23].

The effect of *H. pylori* eradication on dyspeptic symptoms in FD patients has revealed inconclusive results in several studies, both in developed countries and in Asia. [26, 27, 28, 29] Dyspeptic patients who are infected with *H. pylori* often have functional dyspepsia rather than peptic ulcer disease, yet the outcome of eradicating *H. pylori* infection may be suboptimal in FD compared with that for established duodenal ulcer disease. [30] Nevertheless, at a population level, a Cochrane systemic review indicated that there was a 10% relative risk reduction of persistent symptoms in the *H. pylori*-eradication group compared to placebo; the number needed to treat to cure one case of dyspepsia was 14. [31] A recent meta-analysis of the Chinese literature showed that dyspepsia symptoms in FD improved after *H. pylori* eradication with an odds ratio of 3.61, suggesting that this infection might have a greater role in Asian than in Western countries. [32] Thus, *H. pylori* eradication overall does improve dyspepsia, particularly in regions with high prevalence.

4. *H. pylori* diagnostic tests in FD

Tests to diagnosis *H pylori* infection are divided into those that are invasive requiring endoscopy versus those that are noninvasive, not requiring endoscopy. The choice of test depends on issues such as cost (variable in each country), availability, clinical situation, prevalence of infection, pretest probability of infection, and presence of confounding factors (eg, the use of PPI and antibiotics) that may influence test results.

a. Noninvasive tests for *H. pylori*

The noninvasive tests available in clinical practice include serologic tests, urea breath tests, and stool antigen tests. The choice of test is important in terms of validity

1. Serological tests

IgM and IgA antibody tests have not proven to be useful clinically, whereas anti–*H pylori* IgG has a better result. anti–*H pylori* IgG usually can be detected by 3-4 weeks after infection. The three mains methods of commercial kits are ELISA ($90–$95/correct diagnosis),, immunochromatography, and Western blotting.

Most serologic tests carries a high sensitivity (~90 to 100%), but variable specificity (under 85-90%). Their positive and negative predicative values depend upon the background prevalence of *H. pylori* infection in the population at risk. In areas where infection is common, a negative test is likely to be a false negative. Conversely, a positive test amongst those in whom *H pylori* is infrequent is more likely to be a false positive. In developed countries with low prevalence of *H. pylori* infection (<20%), for example, a positive serological test signals active infection only about half the time. Hence, serology should be validated locally. Further, antibody tests can remain positive for years after *H pylori* eradication and have limited value to confirm eradication of *H pylori* infection4.

2. Urea breath test (UBT)

The urea breath test provides a reliable noninvasive method for *H pylori* detection with sensitivity and specificity of 88-95% and 95%-100% respectively. [33] Urea breath testing is not only sensitive and specific but has an important advantage to confirm *H pylori* eradication. Following ingestion of 13C- or 14C-urea, *H pylori*-produced urease enzyme that is resident in the stomach hydrolyzes this labeled urea to $^{14}CO_2$ or $^{13}CO_2$, which can be detected in breath samples [34] (fig. 1). The nonradioactive^{13}C (a stable label) test and the radioactive ^{14}C test have received US Food and Drug Administration (FDA) approval for *H pylori* diagnosis. The dose of radiation in the ^{14}C-urea test however is not approved for use in children and pregnant women [4].

3. Fecal *H. pylori* detection

H. pylori in the stomach also appears in the stool, allowing the development of fecal assays: *H pylori* culture, DNA detected by polymerase chain reaction (PCR), or *H pylori* antigen testing. Only stool antigen has proven to be clinical useful with sensitivities and specificities of more than 90%. Stool antigen assay is advantageous to confirm eradication. To avoid false negative results, it is generally recommended that post-treatment testing with the UBT, histology, stool antigen test or culture be delayed for 4 weeks and the patients should discontinue proton pump inhibitors (PPI) and antibiotic such as amoxicillin, clarithromycin and quinolone groups to ensure that any remaining organisms can repopulate the stomach [4].

b. Invasive tests

Invasive testing which requires endoscopy should be limited to patients who require endoscopy for diagnostic or therapeutic evaluation. Invasive tests available in clinical practice include: gastric biopsies for culture (fig. 2A), gram stain (fig. 2B), histology (fig. 3A), or rapid urease testing (fig. 3B). Rapid urease test such as CLO test plus upper GI endoscopy usually cost between 276-502 (average 389) US dollars. *H pylori* culture is the absolute gold standard to diagnose *H. pylori* but culture generally is not available in most hospitals. Good quality laboratories are capable to culture *H. pylori* from gastric biopsies in more than 80% of instances and also offer susceptibility testing such as E-test.

http://dx.doi.org/10.5772/56652

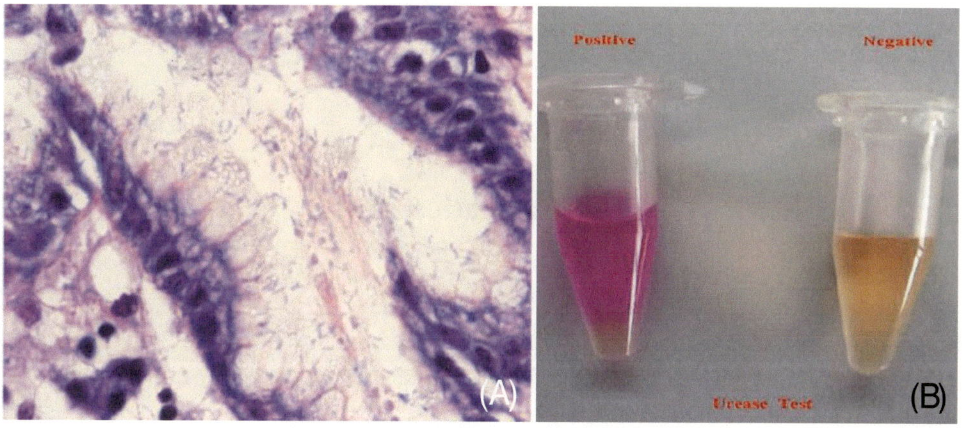

Figure 3. A.) *H pylori* detected by histology; (B.) *H pylori* detected by rapid urease test

Histological examination has an advantage over other diagnostic tests by providing morphological information such as severity of gastritis, and evidence for dysplasia. The accuracy of histological examination however may be variable due to density of *H. pylori* and sampling error, and is dependent upon histopathogical interpretation. The accuracy of histological diagnosis of *H pylori* infection can be improved by adequate biopsies from the antrum and body and by special staining such as a silver staining and the Diff-Quik stain [35].

Rapid urease tests contain a solution or gel with urea and a pH indicator reagent. The presence of urease from *H pylori* results in hydrolysis of neutral urea to alkaline ammonia, which is then visualized by a change in color of the pH indicator. The rapid urease test has a high sensitivity (95%) and specificity (95%), [36] making it an excellent primary diagnostic test.

Any concomitant use of antibiotics or PPI however will reduces bacterial load, and may lead to false negative tests such as rapid urease tests, urea breath test and histology. [4]

4. Test-and-Treat Strategy for *H. pylori*

Proposed strategies based on the noninvasive diagnosis of H. pylori infection so-called "test-and-treat" strategy. This strategy has been proposed for clinical practice in developed countries which has low prevalence of H. pylori infection. Test-and-treat is based on the test of the presence of H. pylori and its subsequent eradication when detected.13 The test-and-scope strategy performing a test to detect H. pylori in all patients and endoscopy only in those who are shown to be infected has been considered useful in clinical practice in some developing countries which has high prevalence of H. pylori infection such as Asia.

5. Management of *H. pylori* infection in FD

Both European (Maastricht IV/ Florence Consensus Report) and Asian consensus reports endorse *H. pylori* testing and eradication as a key management strategy for patients with dyspepsia to produce long-term relief of symptoms. [37,38]

6. Antibiotics use for *H. pylori* eradication

6.1. Amoxicillin

Amoxicillin is a popular antibiotic for treating *H pylori* infection because it is inexpensive and well tolerated, while resistance is rare. [39, 40] Amoxicillin acts by inhibiting the synthesis of the bacterial cell wall and can act locally when delivered into the gastric lumen and systemically once absorbed into the bloodstream. Amoxicillin is pH-dependent; its bactericidal activity increases as the pH rises. As a single agent antibiotic use is not capable of curing *H. pylori* infection, amoxicillin must be combined with other antibiotics such as clarithromycin and metronidazole. [4]

6.2. Clarithromycin

Clarithromycin, a 14-membered ring macrolide antibiotic, is a derivative of erythromycin, sharing a close spectrum and clinical application. Clarithromycin is one of the most acid-stable macrolide with a low minimum inhibitory concentration (MIC) for *H. pylori* treatment. The antimicrobial activity results from its binding to bacterial ribosomes and disrupting bacterial proteinsynthesis. [4] Currently, Clarithromycin resistance is increasing and resulting in a marked reduction in treatment success. [4, 8, 41] Increasing the clarithromycin dosage does not overcome the problem of resistance. This antibiotic frequently causes a bitter taste that causes some patients will stop treatment.

6.3. Metronidazole

Metronidazole is a nitroimidazole group, which is toxic to microaerophilic organisms. Metronidazole is secreted into gastric juice and saliva, and is active after absorption with a half-life of 8 to 12 hours. [4] Metronidazoleis is a pH-independent. [42] After entry into the bacterial cell, metronidazole changes into a toxic form that alters the bacterial enzymes required for transformation. Unlike clarithromycin, metronidazole resistance can be overcome by increasing the dosage. The side effects of short-term use of metronidazole include interactions with alcohol (disulfiram like effect) and gastrointestinal symptoms such as nausea and vomiting. [4]

6.4. Tetracycline

Tetracycline, a derivative of polycyclic naphtacenecarboxamides, is a fine anti–*H. pylori* antimicrobial because it is inexpensive and pH-independent. [4] Tetracycline inhibits bacterial protein synthesis and seems to act luminal or locally. [43] The site of action of tetracycline is the bacterial ribosome, resulting in the interruption of protein biosynthesis. This antibiotic should not be given to pregnant women or children because it causes permanent staining of developing teeth. [4]

6.5. Fluoroquinolones

Fluoroquinolones have been used more popularly for *H pylori* treatment. These drugs block DNA gyrase and DNA synthesis in the organism. Resistance to fluoroquinolones develops rapidly, so that prior use of these medications is associated with a significant rate of resistance. [4]

6.6. Furazolidone

Furazolidone is a monoamine oxidase inhibitor with widely antibacterial activity based on interference with bacterial enzymes. This antibiotic has proven to be an effective part of triple therapy while the development of resistance is rare. Furazolidone is an underused antimicrobial. [44]

6.7. Rifabutin

Rifabutin is a semisynthetic ansamycin antibiotic with low MIC level for *H pylori* infection. This antibiotic is becoming more common and primarily used in combination with PPI and amoxicillin. [4] Rifabutin-based triple therapy for 10 days has been tested as salvage therapy and found to have high eradication rate of over 80%. Ritabutin can have cross-resistance with antimycobacterium. [8]

6.8. Other antimicrobial agent

Bismuth compounds are topically active pH-independent antimicrobial drugs that disrupt the integrity of bacterial cell walls. Bismuth is directly bactericidal, even though its MIC is high for *H pylori.* Bismuth is available in two forms (bismuth subsalicylate and bismuth subcitrate), which have equivalent effect as anti–*H pylori* therapy. *H pylori* resistance has not been reported for this agent. [4]

Regimens available

In recent years, the efficacy of legacy triple therapy for *H. pylori* eradication has declined worldwide to an unacceptable level. The average success rate of triple therapy has also declined to about 70%. [4, 8, 41] Bismuth-based quadruple therapy containing metronidazole is more effective than triple therapy with overall eradication rate of 83% and the eradication rate is higher in metronidazole sensitive group than those of the resistant group. [45] A recent study from Thailand demonstrated that a ten-day sequential therapy is highly effective for *H. pylori* infection with eradication rate of 95% but its efficacy affected by clarithromycin resistance. [41] A study from concomitant therapy evaluated and compared the efficacy of 10-day and 5-day therapy for *H. pylori* eradication using PPI with three antibiotics and found that 10-

day regimen is highly effective with eradication rate of 96% and the 5-day regimen yielded eradication rate of 88%. [46] The available treatment regimens was summarized in table 1. [4]

Legacy therapies
Triple therapy: A PPI plus amoxicillin, 1 g , plus clarithromycin, 500 mg, or metronidazole/tinidazole, 500 mg, twice a day for 14 days
Quadruple therapy: Bismuth, metronidazole, 500 mg, tetracycline, 500 mg, three times a day plus a PPI twice a day for 14 days
Concomitant triple therapies
A PPI plus amoxicillin, 1 g, plus clarithromycin, 500 mg, and metronidazole/tinidazole, 500 mg, twice a day for 14 days
Sequential therapy
A PPI plus 1 g amoxicillin, twice a day for 5 days. On day 6 stop amoxicillin and add clarithromycin, 250 or 500 mg and metronidazole/tinidazole, 500 mg, twice a day to complete the 10-day course.

Table 1. Treatment regimens for *Helicobacter pylori* infections[4]

There are many factors that could influence the eradication rate of *H. pylori*. Compliance is a major concern and how to make the regimen conveniently used by all patients is important. Impact of drug metabolism and CYP2C19 on eradication rate is a new point of concern and needs further research to elucidate this question. The choice of a second-line therapy depends on local antibiotic resistance pattern, previous treatment, drug availability and cost. Second-line salvage therapy after primary therapy failure, levofloxacin based triple therapy resulted in eradication rate of over 80% in patients after failed triple therapy. The accumulation eradication rate after first-line and second-line therapy becomes nearly 90%. This regimen is convenient and well-tolerated but antibiotic resistance to levofloxacin needs to be monitored. Rifabutin-based triple therapy for 10 days has been tested as salvage therapy and found to have high eradication rate of over 80%. Ritabutin can have cross-resistance with antimyco-bacterium. Furazotidone can also be used as salvage therapy but the use is limited by its availability. The summarized efficacy of *H. pylori* treatment regimens is: [8]

- Triple therapy containing PPI plus amoxicillin and clarithromycin or metronidazole has limited efficacy for *H. pylori* eradication with expected eradication rate of 70%.
- Sequential therapy and concomitant therapy yield high eradication rate of over 90% and could be used as first - line therapy.
- Bismuth based quadruple therapy could be used as alternative first - line therapy with high eradication rate.
- Levofloxacin based- triple therapy and concomitant therapy can be used as a second line salvage therapy after failed first - line therapy.

http://dx.doi.org/10.5772/56652

Author details

Ratha-korn Vilaichone and Varocha Mahachai

*Address all correspondence to: vilaichone@yahoo.com

GI Unit, Faculty of Medicine, Thammasat University Hospital, Thailand

References

[1] Goodwin CS, Worsley BW. Microbiology of *Helicobacter pylori*. *Gastroenterol Clin North Am* 1993; 22(1):5-19.

[2] Marshall BJ, Warren JR. Unidentified curved bacilli in the stomach of patients with gastritis and peptic ulceration. *Lancet* 1984; 1: 1311–5.

[3] Atherton JC. The clinical relevance of strain type of *Helicobacter pylori*. *Gut* 1997; 40:701-3.

[4] Vilaichone RK, Mahachai V, Graham DY. *Helicobacter pylori*: Diagnosis and management. *Gastroenterol Clin North Am* 2006; 35(2):229-47.

[5] Tack J, Talley NJ, Camilleri M, *et al*. Functional gastroduodenal disorders. Gastroenterology 2006; 130: 1466–79.

[6] O'Connor H, Sebastian S. The burden of Helicobacter pylori infection in Europe. Aliment Pharmacol Ther 2003; 18 (Suppl. 3): 38–44.

[7] Vilaichone RK, Mahachai V, Tumwasorn S, et al. Molecular epidemiology and outcome of infection *Helicobacter pylori* in Thailand. *Helicobacter* 2004; 9(5): 453-9.

[8] Mahachai V, Vilaichone RK. Current Status of *Helicobacter pylori* Infection in Thailand. *Helicobacter Research* 2011; 15(3): 38-44.

[9] Vilaichone RK, Mahachai V. Current management of *Helicobacter pylori* infection. *J Med Assoc Thai* 2001; 84(Suppl 1): S32-8.

[10] Ghoshal UC, Singh R, Chang F-Y, Hou X, Wong BCY, Kachintorn U. Epidemiology of uninvestigated and functional dyspepsia in Asia: facts and fiction. *J. Neurogastroenterol. Motil*2011; 17: 235–44.

[11] Li XB, Liu WZ, Ge ZZ *et al*. Analysis of clinical characteristics of dyspeptic symptoms in Shanghai patients. *Chin. J. Dig. Dis* 2005;6: 62–7.

[12] Kwan AC, Bao TN, Chakkaphak S *et al*. Validation of Rome IIcriteria for functional gastrointestinal disorders by factor analysis of symptoms in Asian patient sample. *J. Gastroenterol. Hepatol.* 2003;18: 796–802.

[13] Gisbert JP, Pajares JM. Helicobacter pylori "test-and-treat" strategy for dyspeptic patients. *Scand J Gastroenterol* 1999; 34: 644–652.

[14] Lambert JR. The role of *Helicobacter pylori* in nonulcer dyspepsia. A debate—for. *Gastroenterol. Clin. North Am* 1993; 22:141–51.

[15] Jaakkimainen RL, Boyle E, Tudiver F. Is *Helicobacter pylori*associated with non-ulcer dyspepsia and will eradication improvesymptoms? A meta-analysis. *BMJ* 1999; 319: 1040–4.

[16] El-Omar E, Penman I, Ardill JE, McColl KE. A substantial proportion of non-ulcer dyspepsia patients have the same abnormality of acid secretion as duodenal ulcer patients. *Gut* 1995; 36: 534–8.

[17] Vilaichone RK, Mahacahai VM, Tumwasorn S, Kachintorn U. *CagA* genotype and Metronidazole resistant strain of *Helicobacter pylori* in Functional dyspepsia in Thailand. *J Gastroenterol Hepatol* 2011 ;26 Suppl 3:46-8.

[18] Blaser MJ, Perez-Perez GI, Kleanthous H., et al. Infection with *Helicobacter pylori* strains possessing *cagA* is associated with an increased risk of developing adenocarcinoma of the stomach. *Cancer Res*1995: 55(10); 2111–15.

[19] Yamaoka Y, Orito E, Mizokami M., et al. *Helicobacter pylori* in North and South America before Columbus. *FEBS Lett* 2002: 517(1-3):180-4.

[20] Yamaoka Y, Ojo O, Fujimoto S., et al. *Helicobacter pylori* outer membrane proteins and gastroduodenal disease. *Gut* 2006: 55; 775–781.

[21] Taneike I, Nami A, O'Connor A, et al. Analysis of drug resistance and virulence-factor genotype of Irish *Helicobacter pylori* strains: is there any relationship between resistance to metronidazole and cagA status? *Aliment Pharmacol Ther* 2009 Oc;30(7): 784-90

[22] Vilaichone RK, Mahachai V, Tumwasorn S, et al. Outcome of *Helicobacter pylori* Infections in Relation to Gastric Mucosal Cytokines Levels, Interluekin-1 Polymorphisms and *cagA* Genotypes. *Scan J Gastroenerol* 2005; 40: 530-39.

[23] Suzuki T, Matsuo K, Sawaki A et al. Systematic review and meta-analysis: importance of CagA status for successful eradication of Helicobacter pylori infection. *Aliment Pharmacol Ther* 2006: 24(2):273–280.

[24] Atherton JC, Tham KT, Peek RM Jr, et al. Density of *Helicobacter pylori* infection in vivo as assessed by quantitative culture and histology. *J Infect Dis* 1996; 174: 552–6.

[25] Hamlet A, Thoreson AC, Nilsson O, et al. Duodenal *Helicobacter pylori* infection differs in cagA genotype between asymptomatic subjects and patients with duodenal ulcers. *Gastroenterology* 1999; 116:259–68

[26] Moayyedi P, Soo S, Deeks J *et al*. Systematic review and economic evaluation of *Helicobacter pylori* eradication treatment for non-ulcer dyspepsia. *BMJ* 2000; 321: 659–64.

[27] Laine L, Schoenfeld P, Fennerty MB. Therapy for *Helicobacterpylori* in patients with nonulcer dyspepsia. A meta-analysis of randomized, controlled trials. *Ann. Intern. Med* 2001; 134:361–9.

[28] Kawamura A, Adachi K, Takashima T *et al*. Prevalence of functional dyspepsia and its relationship with *Helicobacter pylori* infection in a Japanese population. *J. Gastroenterol. Hepatol* 2001;16: 384–8.

[29] Miwa H, Hirai S, Nagahara A *et al*. Cure of *Helicobacter pylori*infection does not improve symptoms in non-ulcer dyspepsia patients-a double-blind placebo-controlled study. *Alimen Pharmacol Ther* 2000; 14: 317–24.

[30] Wong WM, Xiao SD, Hu PJ *et al*. Standard treatment for *Helicobacter pylori* infection is suboptimal in non-ulcer dyspepsia compared with duodenal ulcer in Chinese. *Aliment Pharmacol Ther* 2005; 21: 73–81.

[31] Moayyedi P, Soo S, Deeks J *et al*. Eradication of *Helicobacter pylori* for non-ulcer dyspepsia. *Cochrane Database Syst. Rev.* 2006;(2): CD002096.

[32] Jin X, Li YM. Systematic review and meta-analysis from Chinese literature: the association between *Helicobacter pylori* eradication and improvement of functional dyspepsia. *Helicobacter* 2007; 12:541–6.

[33] *Howden CW, Hunt RH.* Guidelines for the management of *Helicobacter pylori* infection. Ad Hoc Committee on Practice Parameters of the American College of Gastroenterology. *Am J Gastroenterol 1998;93(12): 2330-8.*

[34] Vaira D, Malfertheiner P, Megraud F, et al. Diagnosis of *Helicobacter pylori* infection with a new non-invasive antigen-based assay. HpSA European study group. *Lancet* 1999;354(9172):30–3.

[35] El-Zimaity HM, Segura AM, Genta RM, et al. Histologic assessment of Helicobacter pylori status after therapy: comparison of Giemsa, Diff-Quik, and Genta stains. *Mod Pathol* 1998;11(3):288–91.

[36] HowdenCW, Hunt RH. Guidelines for the management of Helicobacter pylori infection. AdHoc Committee on Practice Parameters of the American College of Gastroenterology. *Am J Gastroenterol* 1998;93(12):2330–8.

[37] Malfertheiner P, Megraud F, O'Morain CA,et al. Management of Helicobacter pylori infection--the Maastricht IV/ Florence Consensus Report. Gut 2012;61(5):646-64.

[38] Miwa H, Ghoshal UC, Fock KM, et al. Asian Consensus Report on Functional Dyspepsia. J Gastroenterol Hepatol 2012; 27(4):626-41.

[39] Duck WM, Sobel J, Pruckler JM, et al. Antimicrobial resistance incidence and risk factors among Helicobacter pylori-infected persons, United States. *Emerg Infect Dis* 2004;10(6):1088–94.

[40] Watanabe K, Tanaka A, Imase K, et al. Amoxicillin resistance in Helicobacter pylori: studies from Tokyo, Japan from 1985 to 2003. *Helicobacter* 2005; 10(1):4–11.

[41] Mahachai V, Sirimontaporn N, Tumwasorn S, et al. Sequential Therapy in Clarithromycin Sensitive and Resistant *H. pylori* Based on PCR Molecular Test. *J Gastroenterol Hepatol* 2011; 26(5):825-8.

[42] van Zanten SJ, Goldie J, Hollingsworth J, et al. Secretion of intravenously administered antibiotics in gastric juice: implications for management of *Helicobacter pylori*. *J Clin Pathol* 1992; 45(3):225–7.

[43] Tytgat GN. Treatments that impact favorably upon the eradication of Helicobacter pylori and ulcer recurrence. *Aliment Pharmacol Ther* 1994;8(4):359–68.

[44] Segura AM, Gutierrez O, OteroW, et al. Furazolidone, amoxycillin, bismuth triple therapy for Helicobacter pylori infection. *Aliment Pharmacol Ther* 1997;11(3):529–32.

[45] Mahachai V, Treeprasertsuk S, Chaithongrat S, Vilaichone RK. Seven day Bismuth-based quadruple therapy as an initial therapy for *Helicobacter pylori* infection in a high Metroninazole resistant area. *Helicobacter* 2007; 12(4) (A).

[46] Kongchayanun C,Vilaichone RK, Pornthisarn B, et al. Pilot studies to identify the optimum duration of concomitant *Helicobacter pylori* eradication therapy in Thailand. *Helicobacter* 2012; 17(4):282-5.

Chapter 5

Helicobacter pylori—Associated Dyspepsia in Paediatrics

Mónica Roxo-Rosa, Mónica Oleastro and
Ana Isabel Lopes

Additional information is available at the end of the chapter

http://dx.doi.org/10.5772/56551

1. Introduction

Helicobacter pylori ubiquitously infects the human gastric mucosa since time immemorial, predictably before the man's diaspora out of East Africa around 58,000 years ago [1]. Colonization may have been somehow beneficial for human carriers, allowing the co-evolution of this gram-negative bacterium and its host over the centuries. Yet, at least nowadays [2], this may not be a peaceful association, with infection almost invariably causing an acute host immune response. However, in a fully adapted manner, *H. pylori* avoids recognition and, thus, clearance, by the host immune system, with both infection and the consequent gastritis persisting throughout the patients' life. The clinical outcome of this persistence is dependent on a sophisticated crosstalk between the host and the pathogen. If often asymptomatic, the *H. pylori*-associated non-ulcer dyspepsia is clearly the strongest aetiological factor for severe gastric diseases that will develop late in adult life in a minority of infected patients, *i.e.*, peptic ulcer disease, both gastric and duodenal ulcers, and gastric cancer, namely, adenocarcinoma and mucosa associated lymphoid tissue (MALT) lymphoma *(reviewed in [3])*. Peptic ulcer disease rarely occurs soon after *H. pylori* infection [4-8] that generally starts in childhood; this presumably reflects marked differences in the virulence [9-16] and/or in the susceptibility of young patients [17-19].

This chapter, focussing on the paediatric population, seeks to explore: the prevalence of *H. pylori* infection; the molecular mechanism used by *H. pylori* during colonization and infection; the role of this bacterium in the development of peptic ulcer-related organic dyspepsia; and the genetic/proteome profile of the *H. pylori*-strains associated with peptic ulcer disease.

1.1. Prevalence of infection

H. pylori is one of the most common gastrointestinal bacterial infections among humans, affecting more than 50% of the world's population [1,20]. *Infection is usually acquired during the first years of life in both developing and industrialized countries, with* intra-familial spread playing a central role in transmission of the infection [21,22]. The prevalence of *H. pylori* is markedly variable between developing and developed countries, and even among individuals living in the same country, varying according to ethnicity, place of birth and socioeconomic factors. Besides geographic area, age is also significantly and independently associated with an increase in *H. pylori* prevalence, a phenomenon known as birth cohort effect, which is a progressive reduction of the infection rate in successive birth cohorts, due to the improvements in general living conditions (reviewed in [23]). In less developed countries the infection rate reaches almost 50% in very young children and more than 90% in adults, whereas in industrialized countries *H. pylori* infects 20-50% of adults and less than 10% of children, and has been declining over time [23,24]. Indeed, the prevalence of *H. pylori* infection is *showing a decreased trend* worldwide that *is directly associated with an improvement in the socioeconomic status and hygienic conditions of the populations.*

Accordingly, *in Europe and North America, the epidemiology of H. pylori infection in children has changed in recent decades. Nowadays, low incidence rates are found in the northern and western European countries, resulting in prevalence far below 10% in children and adolescents. In contrast, the infection is still common in certain geographic areas such as southern or eastern Europe, Mexico, and certain immigrant populations from South America, Africa, most Asian countries, and first-nation (aboriginal) people in North America* [25-27]. In Portugal with the worst scenario of Europe, the prevalence of H. pylori infection is closer to the situation observed in developing countries, reaching 80% among the adult population in their early nineties, and, more recently, varying from approximately 20% in young children (less than 5 years old) to 50% in children 10 to 15 years old [28,29].

The absence of effective vaccines [30] and of efficient alternatives to antibiotics [31-34] renders difficult the worldwide prevention of *H. pylori* infection-associated diseases through massive eradication of the bacterium. The current antibiotic therapy against *H. pylori* infection fails in about 20% of the patients; depending on the therapeutic schema and strain resistance pattern, the failure rate may reach 70%. Antibiotic resistance, mainly to clarithromycin, is the major factor affecting the efficacy of standard triple therapy of *H. pylori* infection (co-administration of two antibiotics and a proton pump inhibitor or ranitidine bismuth for seven to ten days). In fact, the resistance rates to this and other second line antibiotics, such as the fluoroquinolones, are increasing in many geographical areas [34-36].

Several studies reveal a similar or higher resistance rate to clarithromycin among paediatric isolates as compared to those obtained from adults, especially in southern European countries, reflecting the recognized overuse of macrolides in children in these countries [31,34,37,38]. As an example, Portugal displays one of the highest rates of *H. pylori* primary resistance to clarithromycin in Europe, similarly high in children as among adults (≈33%) [34]. Moreover, resistance to second line antibiotics has rapidly increased over the last decade and is a matter of concern [31-34]. This places the research on disease-specific bacterial biomarkers and their associated molecular mechanisms as a top priority to define disease-risk and to target *H. pylori* eradication in high-risk individuals. Ultimately, it may provide novel bacterial and/or host's therapeutic or vaccine targets.

1.2. Molecular mechanisms of *H. pylori* colonization and infection

1.2.1. Acid resistance and motility

In a fully adapted manner, during colonization and persistence, this neutralophile bacterium resists gastric acidity mainly through its urease activity. Its urease enzyme, a Ni^{2+}-containing dodecameric protein of approximately 1100 kDa, composed of 12 small subunits, UreA (27 kDa), and 12 large subunits, UreB (62 kDa), catalyzes the hydrolysis of urea into ammonia and carbon dioxide, buffering both the bacteria cytoplasm and periplasm [39]. Accounting for 5-10% of the total protein content, urease is one of the most abundant proteins in the *H. pylori* proteome [16,30]. Probably due to the toxicity of ammonia, urease activity is known to be dependent on low pH and/or Ni^{2+} concentration conditions [39,40], being essential for bacteria survival only under acidic conditions. In the early stages of colonization, *H. pylori* seeks parts of the stomach with higher pH, such as the antrum (the distal part of the stomach). Indeed, this bacterium uses the pH gradient as chemotactic signal to achieve regions of neutral pH, since its spatial orientation is lost in the absence of the mucus pH gradient [41]. Thus, the acid-producing parietal cells may protect the corpus region from initial invasion.

Efficient colonization of the gastric niche by *H. pylori* is also dependent on how fast it escapes from the lumen of the stomach and reaches the mucus layer, avoiding elimination by gastric peristalsis [42]. Its helical shape and the two to six polar, sheathed flagella provide swimming abilities. According to a longstanding theory [43], the helical shape allows *H. pylori* to have a corkscrew motion which, although not being essential for motility, enhances its ability to swim through the viscous mucus layer. The machinery that gives rise to the spiral shape of this bacterium remains largely unknown, but seems dependent on the coordinated action of multiple proteins in a shape-generating pathway that leads to the relaxation of the peptidoglycan crosslinking [44]. Flagella are, however, essential for *H. pylori* motility. Indeed, aflagellated strains (obtained by elimination of both *flaA* and *flaB*, genes encoding the two major components of flagellar filament, flagellins A and B) [45], as well as strains presenting non-functional flagella (in knockout *motB* models lacking the gene that encodes the MotB flagellar motor protein), are non-motile [42]. Such mutants are able to establish only transient colonization in animal models [42,46]. Moreover, lower-motility strains are long known to induce *in vitro* reduced inflammation levels, when compared to higher motility strains [47]. Once in the mucus layer of the stomach, *H. pylori* resides here thereafter, either freely swimming [43] or attached to host's extracellular mucins [41], getting closer to the host's gastric epithelial surface whenever necessary. Occasionally *H. pylori* also can be internalized, entering the gastric epithelial cells [48]. Invasion beyond the epithelial layer is, however, is a rare event.

1.2.2. Bacterial Adherence

In the human stomach, the vast majority of *H. pylori* cells exist in their motile form within the mucus layer lining; only a small portion (≈30%) are adherent to the surfaces of epithelial cells [41]. Nevertheless, adherence to the gastric epithelium is important for the ability of *H. pylori* to cause disease because this intimate attachment facilitates: 1) persistence, by preventing the bacteria from being eliminated from the stomach through mucus turnover and gastric peristalsis, and also by enabling the bacteria to replicate; 2) evasion from the human immune system; 3) efficient delivery of the bacterial toxic proteins; and 4) acquiring nutrients released from the damaged host cells.

H. pylori expresses a multitude of different adhesins. Best characterized is the blood group antigen-binding adhesin (BabA), a ligand of ABO (of the blood group system) Lewis b (Le^b) antigens [49]. Sequence analyses reveals the existence of two allelic variants of *babA*, the *babA1* and *babA2* alleles, which are identical except for a 10 base pair insertion that results in a translational initiation codon present in *babA2* but absent in *babA1*, and of a highly homologous gene, *babB*. Of these, only *babA2* allele encodes a functional Le^b adhesin [49]. BabA is not likely to be essential for the colonization; BabA-expressing strains are no different in this step compared to BabA-non-expressing strains [50]. BabA, being an adhesin, however likely plays an important role in the induction of host inflammatory response. Indeed, *babA2* allele is clinically important, namely in a *vacA/cagA*-positive genetic background (two additional important virulence factors discussed in section 1.2.3. of this chapter), which is associated with peptic ulcer disease and gastric cancer [51]. BabA-expressing strains induces change in the glycosylation pattern of the gastric mucosa of humans and animal models [50].

The second best characterized *H. pylori* adhesin is the sialic acid binding adhesin (SabA) which mediates attachment to the inflammation-associated (sialylated $Lewis^x$ and $Lewis^a$) antigens [52]. In fact, gastric tissue inflammation and malignant transformation promote synthesis of sialylated glycoconjugates, which are rare in healthy human stomachs [52, 53]. Accordingly, high levels of sialylated glycoconjugates are found in *H. pylori* infected persons; these decrease after eradication of the infection and resolution of the gastritis [54]. *H. pylori* can agglutinate erythrocytes and neutrophils *in vitro*. The SabA adhesin is the hemagglutinin of *H. pylori* and allows bacterial adherence to blood cells; this may result in systemic dissemination of the pathogen [55]. Moreover, the binding of SabA to sialic acid carries neutrophil receptors, essential for the nonopsonic activation of human neutrophils [56]. Neutrophils play a major role in the epithelium injury, since these cells have direct toxic effects on the epithelial cells, through the induction of an oxidative burst, with the release of reactive oxygen and nitrogen species. Thus, the neutrophil activating capacity of SabA makes this protein an additional virulence factor that is important in the pathogenesis of *H. pylori* infection.

The outer membrane inflammatory protein (OipA), a member of the Hop family of proteins, is another *H. pylori* membrane protein with an active role in bacterial adherence, for which no host receptors are known. Its encoding gene (*oipA*) is present in all *H. pylori* strains but it is only expressed in those presenting the *oipA* "on" (*i.e.*, functional) genotype. This is regulated by slipped-strand mispairing, depending on the number of CT repeats in the 5′ region of the gene [57]. OipA expression by *H. pylori* is associated with high bacterial densities, severe neutrophil infiltration and, ultimately, with peptic ulceration and gastric cancer [58,59]. Supporting the later association, the inactivation of *oipA* results in a reduced nuclear translocation of β-catenin, a known factor involved in the transcriptional up-regulation of genes implicated in carcinogenesis [59].

1.2.3. Delivery and virulence factors

After adherence, *H. pylori* delivers its virulence factors into the cytoplasm of the host's cells by using a type IV secretion system (T4SS) and/or outer membrane vesicles. The genes encoding the components of the T4SS, which is a syringe-like pilus protruding from the bacterial surface used to inject virulence factors in host target cells' cytoplasm, are located in the *cag* pathogenicity island (PAI) [60]. This is an approximately 40 kpb chromosomal insertion that is thought to have been incorporated into the *H. pylori* genome by horizontal transfer from an unknown source [61]. As a result, strains are heterogenic regarding the presence of this chromosomal region, varying between those that contain the intact *cag* PAI to those that completely lack it. For those lacking an intact T4SS, the delivery of their virulence factors is totally dependent on the secretion of outer membrane vesicles with a still poorly known content; these are endocytosed by the host epithelial cells (reviewed in [62]).

Encoded by *cytotoxin associated gene A*, one of the 32 genes of the *cag* PAI region, CagA is perhaps the most extensively studied translocated protein, the only known effector protein injected by the T4SS. Once injected into cytoplasm of target cells, CagA interferes with several host cell signalling cascades, ultimately inducing abnormal proliferation, cytoskeleton rearrangements and inflammation through the release of cytokines, such as interleukin-1β (IL-1β), IL-8 and tumour necrosis factor-α (TNF-α) (reviewed in [63]). There are two types of clinical isolates regarding CagA: those producing this protein (*cagA*-positive *H. pylori* strains), and the CagA-nonproducing strains (*cagA*-negative *H. pylori* strains). The *cagA*-positive strains are considerably more virulent [60]. In Western countries, individuals carriers of *cagA*-positive strains are thus at higher risk of peptic ulcer disease and/or gastric cancer [64,65], leading to the classification of CagA as a bacterium-derived oncogenic protein [66]. In a not fully undisclosed manner, the virulence of the *cagA*-positive strains is associated with the number and the type of the phosphorylation motifs of the C-terminal variable region of the protein. Of these motifs, defined as EPIYA (Glu-Pro-Ile-Tyr-Ala) A, B, C and D according to different flanking amino acids, CagA protein nearly always possesses EIPYA-A and B segments, followed by none, one, two or three C segments in Western-strains or a D segment in strains of East Asian countries. The East Asian-type of CagA (ABD) is known to be more carcinogenic than the Western-type; within the latter, the variants possessing multiple EPIYA-C motifs (ABCC or ABCCC) are more virulent compared with those with a single segment (ABC) (reviewed in [63]). Moreover, the association of CagA expression levels with polymorphisms in the *cagA* promoter region may further contribute to differences in virulence among *cagA*-positive strains and different disease-associated risks [67]. The virulence of the strain must also be dependent on additional bacterial factors, since in East Asia most strains are *cagA*-positive irrespective of the patient disease.

The vacuolating toxin (VacA), another important virulence factor (reviewed in [68]), is synthesized as a pro-toxin of ≈140 kDa, which contains a *N*-terminal signal sequence, a passenger domain and *C*-terminal autotransporter domain. The passenger toxin domain (≈88 kDa) is cleaved and processed at some point during its secretion into the extracellular milieu through the autotransporter that functions as a type V secretion system. This 88 kDa toxin is further proteolytically cleaved, creating a *N*-terminal fragment of ≈33 kDa (p33) and a *C*-terminal fragment of ≈55 kDa (p55) that remain non-covalently associated. Required for the cytotoxic activity, the p33 subunit is postulated to be involved in the formation of anionic membrane channels, while p55 subunit seems to mediate VacA binding to host cells (reviewed in [68]). These functions are, however, highly dependent of the tridimensional structure of both subunits [69,70]. Once secreted by the bacterial cells, VacA triggers various responses in the host, resulting in the cellular vacuolation, pore formation in the cell membrane, disruption of endosomal/lysosomal structure and function, apoptosis by toxin trafficking to mitochondria, and immunomodulation [71-73]. Virtually all *H. pylori* strains have a functional VacA. However, the amount of toxin produced is related to the allelic variation of the encoding gene, especially in its signal and middle regions (reviewed in [74]). Therefore, an association between particular *vacA* allele types and peptic ulcer disease has been reported worldwide..

The ancient association between *H. pylori* and the modern humans [1,20] has determined the abnormal high diversity in both their genetic background and the virulence observed among strains. This generates complex scenario that creates difficulty in understanding the contribution of each individual factor. Nevertheless, *H. pylori* strains presenting the association of these two virulence factors, *i.e.*, *cagA*-positive and *vacA*-toxigenic alleles, are considered to be more virulent and thus more associated with severe organic dyspepsia inducers of a high production of proinflammatory cytokines in the gastric mucosa and thus more severe non-ulcer dyspepsia. Even so, these virulence factors do not appear to determine the overall pattern of gastroduodenal disease and a complex interplay between host bacterial factors and environment seems to be involved in the development of gastric pathology [75].

1.2.4. Evasion

Upon colonization, *H. pylori*-infected patients experience a strong and complex immune response in the gastric mucosa, both at the humoral and cellular levels; despite this response, nevertheless the infection fails to clear. Therefore, in the absence of effective treatment, infection becomes chronic, persists, and contributes to the immunopathology. The persistence of infection throughout the life of its host is guaranteed by a set of molecular mechanisms used by *H. pylori* to constantly evade the host immune response (reviewed in [76]). Bacterial mimicry and genetic diversity play a central role in such successful strategies.

Mimicking the cell surfaces of the host, the lipopolysaccharide of the *H. pylori* cell wall is relatively anergic compared to other gram-negative bacteria. In fact, the variable part of the *O*-antigen chain of *H. pylori* lipopolysaccharide is composed of host-related Lewis antigens, making it unrecognizable to the host immune system [77]. Therefore, this pathogen not only binds to human Lewis antigens through BabA and SabA, but it also expresses Lewis-like antigens facilitating the escape from the host immune system. Another ingenious camouflage

http://dx.doi.org/10.5772/56551

used by *H. pylori* is the expression of proteins at its surface, which specifically bind to host-secreted proteins, *e.g.*, bacterial plasminogen-binding proteins (PgbA and PgbB). This allows the bacterium to be coated with host proteins [78]. *H. pylori* also avoids immune recognition through the *in vitro* and *in vivo* impairment of the expression of host's specific heat shock proteins, thus, inactivating both the innate and adaptive immune response [79].

Allelic diversification of its virulence factors encoding genes allows *H. pylori* to occupy different microenvironments within the human stomach and to adapt to the varying conditions in the niche over time. This is even more efficient, considering that the expression of different variants of those genes may switch through mechanisms of phase variation. Indeed, several *in vitro* studies have demonstrated that *H. pylori* Lewis-like antigens can undergo phase variation (reviewed in [76]). Moreover, in animal models, persistent infection leads to the loss of expression of *babA*. This occurs either by phase variation switching between an "on" and an "off" status in a manner similar to that described for *oipA* (see section 1.2.2 of this chapter), or by nonreciprocal gene conversion of *babA* to *babB* [80].

The existence of a small subpopulation of *H. pylori* within gastric epithelial cells (as briefly discussed in section 1.2.1 of this chapter) may represent a sanctuary site that protects bacteria against immune clearance [48].

1.3. Peptic Ulcer — Related organic dyspepsia in paediatrics, a rare event

Although rarely associated with severe forms of organic dyspepsia (namely peptic ulcer disease) in the paediatric age group, *H. pylori* is clearly linked with acute gastric inflammation in childhood and occurs frequently in children with dyspepsia [81]. This important association gains relevance when considering that: a) gastric colonization by *H. pylori* occurring in childhood and the consequent inflammation continues for life if left untreated; and b) *this* lifelong persistence of inflammation after decades of infection is the main etiology for peptic ulceration and/or cancer in adulthood. Moreover, some studies suggest a possible impact of *H. pylori*-associated dyspepsia on anthropometry, as children with dyspepsia and *H. pylori* infection are shorter and lighter than children with similar symptoms but no infection [82,83].

Evidence for the importance of *H. pylori* infection as a factor for dyspepsia in childhood comes from *H. pylori* eradication resulting in a significant long-term improvement of dyspeptic symptoms [84]. The symptoms of *H. pylori*-associated paediatric dyspepsia however do not differ from those of non-infected dyspeptic children [85], raising questions about which approach should be adopted in children with dyspepsia, in terms of *H. pylori* testing. According to current guidelines for the management of *H. pylori* infection at pediatric age [86,87], the primary goal of diagnostic interventions should be to determine the cause of the presenting gastrointestinal symptoms ("scope and treat" strategy) and not just the presence of *H. pylori* infection ("test and treat" strategy). Indeed, recurrent abdominal pain is not an indication for a "test and treat" strategy concerning *H. pylori* infection in children, as evidence regarding the association with *H. pylori* infection has been so far inconclusive (even in the presence of peptic ulcer). Indeed, several studies using different noninvasive tests for *H pylori* infection compared the prevalence of positive results in children with recurrent abdominal pain and controls and found no significant difference in infection rates between cases and controls [88,89]. On the other hand, pediatric studies are limited by the lack of a clear definition for recurrent abdominal pain or by the use of nonspecific criteria for the diagnosis of chronic abdominal pain [90]. Nevertheless, in patients with persistent abdominal pain (after exclusion of other causes, such as lactose intolerance, giardiasis, celiac disease, *inflammatory bowel disease*, among others) and/ or severe upper abdominal symptoms (namely suggesting peptic ulcer disease, such as nocturnal pain), upper endoscopy with biopsy should be performed (diagnostic investigation of choice). Furthermore, testing for *H. pylori* in children/adolescents should be considered if there is a family history of gastric cancer and in children/adolescents with refractory iron deficiency anemia, when no other cause is found. In these settings, when upper endoscopy is performed, the presence of *H. pylori* should be systematically sought through histological examination and, whenever feasible, culture and antibiotic susceptibility testing; treatment should be offered in the presence of *H. pylori* positivity. Population screening for *H. pylori* in asymptomatic children to prevent gastric cancer is not warranted. Although ^{13}C-urea breath testing is a validated noninvasive diagnostic test for *H. pylori* infection in children, a "test and treat" strategy including this tool should not be indiscriminately adopted in clinical practice at this age group, considering the fact that this test merely identifies *H. pylori* presence but not necessarily the causality of symptoms. Noninvasive tests for *H.pylori* include different methods for the detection of bacterial antigens in stool, detection of antibodies (IgG, IgA) against *H. pylori* in serum, urine, and oral samples, and the ^{13}C-UBT. In the paediatric group, both fecal antigens determination and respiratory test are reliable to determine whether *H pylori* has been eradicated or not after antibiotic treatment, while tests based on the detection of antibodies against *H pylori* are considered not reliable for use in the clinical setting, but may be useful in epidemiological studies [91].

Therefore, *H. pylori infection in childhood differs from adults not only in terms of the prevalence of the infection and a higher rate of antibiotic resistance, but also with respect to the complication rate, age-specific problems with diagnostic tests and drugs, and the near-absence of gastric malignancies* [92]. Nevertheless, H. pylori-associated peptic ulcer disease may also occur shortly after infection in childhood [4-8]. This rare event may be due to more virulent strains [9-16], and/or more predisposed subjects [17-19]. The two forms of H. pylori-associated peptic ulcers, i.e., gastric ulcer and duodenal ulcers, are divergent in prevalence and physiopathology, but both cause considerable patients' morbidity entailing high annual costs of treatment [93].

1.3.1. Prevalence of H. pylori-associated gastric and duodenal ulcers in childhood

In general, about 10-15% of the H. pylori infected patients suffer from duodenal ulcer disease and 2-5% with gastric ulcer and/or gastric cancer late in the adulthood [3]. Population-based studies in patients with organic dyspepsia suggest that peptic ulcer disease related to H. pylori infection is decreasing in prevalence in Western countries, along with a decrease in the prevalence of infection [94]. The former should be a direct consequence of the second; with improved living standards, cohorts of children became progressively less likely to acquire the organism and thus suffer from H. pylori-associated diseases. Nevertheless, specific populations such as immigrants and rural communities may have a high prevalence of infection and peptic ulcer disease; these individuals should be separately reviewed even in areas where the general prevalence of H. pylori infection has declined below 15% [95]. Despite changing prevalence trends, H. pylori-induced gastritis causing mucosal ulceration either in the stomach (gastric ulcer) or the proximal duodenum (duodenal ulcer) is a relatively uncommon event in children, compared with adults [4-8]. In fact, during childhood, H. pylori is associated with predominant antral gastritis or with pangastritis [96]. *In children, few studies have yet investigated the actual trend of H. pylori prevalence in peptic ulcer disease* [5-8] and the available data are more difficult to interpret, considering that the rates of peptic ulcer diagnosis depend also on the clinical setting (endoscopy versus outpatient clinic or hospital admissions) [97,98]. For example, in Italy the detection rate of ulcer disease was 7.8% out of an average of 180 paediatric gastrointestinal endoscopies performed each year [99]. Similarly, a retrospective review (from 1998 to 2006) showed that 43 (6.9%) out of 619 Chinese children who underwent upper endoscopy for investigation of upper gastrointestinal symptoms had peptic ulcer [7]; and another retrospective study (from 2003 to 2006) have also reported a high incidence of peptic ulcer (6.8%) in Israeli children submitted to upper endoscopy [100]. In Canada, however, the approximate incidence of peptic ulcer was 1 case per 2,500 hospital admissions [92]. In a recent large European multicenter study, including 1233 symptomatic children with H. pylori infection, peptic ulcer disease was diagnosed in less than 5% of children younger than 12 years of age and in ≈10% of teenagers [8]. Interestingly, other studies indicate a higher association of H. pylori with peptic ulcer in adolescents than in younger children [100,101]. But, the prevalence of H. pylori-positive ulcers in children also differs between countries and this is not completely explained by the prevalence of the infection in the population studied. This is easily demonstrated from data collected from January 2001 to December 2002 on 518 children from the paediatric European register for treatment of H. pylori [5]. At endoscopy, 454 of those patients had H. pylori-associated gastritis and 64 had a peptic ulcer (12.3%). This series also included children from Russia, who had a significantly higher prevalence of peptic ulcer (35%) compared to that of the remainder of European children (6.7%) [6]. In another report, school-aged children with chronic abdominal complaints living in the rural area of Russia had a high prevalence rate of H. pylori infection (80%) and also of peptic ulcer disease (24%) [102].

In adults, the prevalence of *H. pylori* infection is higher than 95% in duodenal ulcer cases and around 60% to 80% in gastric ulcer cases [103]. This scenario is similar in children i.e. when *H. pylori*-associated ulcers occur in children, duodenal ulceration is much more frequently identified than gastric ulcers [104]. In fact, pooled analysis of early reports (from 1983 to 1994) has demonstrated that the prevalence of *H. pylori* in children with duodenal ulcer was relatively higher (ranging from 33% to 100%, with a median value of 92%), compared with children with gastric ulcer (ranging from 11% to 75%, with a median value of 25%) [104]. A more recent retrospective study (from 1995 to 2001) from Japan confirmed a very high prevalence of *H. pylori* in antral gastritis and duodenal ulcer (98.5% and 83%, respectively), also identifying *H. pylori* as a risk factor for the development of gastric ulcer although with a lower prevalence of infection (less than 50%) [101]. Finally, in a Chinese study, it was reported that among 43 Chinese children suffering with peptic ulcer disease, 37 had duodenal ulcer, of which 21 were *H. pylori* positive, while only six had gastric ulcer, of which only two were positive for the infection [7]. In summary, *H. pylori* infection is much more associated to duodenal ulcer than to gastric ulcer, in both children and adults.

The causative role of *H. pylori* in gastric ulcers in children and adolescents is, therefore, less certain when compared to adults, possibly reflecting the fact that a large proportion of gastric ulcers are secondary in nature in children. Characteristically, in children younger than 10 years of age, peptic ulcers are usually due to noxious agents (such as corticosteroids and non-steroidal anti-inflammatory drugs (NSAIDs)) or occur after major stresses (such as burns, trauma, and systemic illness). In these settings, upper gastrointestinal tract haemorrhage, vomiting and perforation are frequent presenting features. The ulcers tend not to recur after healing. In older children and adolescents, the clinical presentation and natural history of peptic ulcers are similar to that observed in adults, presenting as epigastric and nocturnal abdominal pain and being usually associated with *H. pylori* infection [8,100,101]. In this setting, even though the acute ulcer is likely to heal, the natural history is for ulcer recurrence. Moreover, the complication rate of peptic ulceration is important. The estimated incidence of peptic ulcer bleeding in the US paediatric population also has ranged from 0.5 to 4.4/100,000 individuals in 2008 [105].

These and other differences explain why some of the recommendations for adults may not apply in children [87,96]. Few randomized, placebo-controlled treatment trials are available in children for the different outcomes (gastritis or peptic ulcer), and often consist of only small numbers of cases [86,106]. Clearly in children as in adults, successful eradication of *H. pylori* markedly reduces the risk of ulcer recurrence [107-110]. Thus, there is general consensus worldwide to treat *H. pylori* infection when there is endoscopic evidence of peptic ulceration. Triple therapy is the treatment of choice in children for endoscopically proven duodenal ulcer and histologically proven *H. pylori* antral gastritis [91, 96, 111, 112].

1.3.2. Differences in the physiopathology of H. pylori*-associated gastric and duodenal ulcers*

Peptic ulceration is a multifactorial disease ultimately explained by disequilibrium between aggressive injurious factors and defensive gastroduodenal mucosa-protective factors, which raises the vulnerability of this mucosa to luminal secretions. *H. pylori* infection is considered the major causative factor for peptic ulceration. Nevertheless, there are other injurious mechanisms jeopardizing the mucosal integrity: some viral infections (*e.g.* cytomegalovirus and herpes simplex); drug-induced injury, particularly acetylsalicylic acid, NSAIDs and chemotherapy; vascular disorders interfering with perfusion; major stresses; and syndromes in which a marked overproduction of gastric acid occurs, as is the case of the Zollinger-Ellison syndrome and, more commonly in children, antral G cell hyperplasia (also referred to as pseudo-Zollinger Ellison syndrome) [113].

Although differing in their pathogenesis, both *H. pylori*-associated duodenal ulcers and gastric ulcers are intimately related to changes in the acid production by the gastric mucosa [113, 114]. Indeed, *H. pylori* infection can result in increased, decreased or no overall change in the level of gastric acid secretion. Duodenal ulcers arise on a background of *H. pylori*–induced antral-predominant gastritis with sparing of the oxyntic mucosa, resulting in hypergastrinemia and consequent high levels of acid production from the healthy gastric corpus following meal or hormonal stimulation. In response to the excessive acid secretion, the duodenum develops gastric metaplasia. This, unlike the normal duodenal mucosa, can be colonized by

http://dx.doi.org/10.5772/56551

H. pylori with consequent inflammation and ulceration [113]. Eradication of the *H. pylori* infection corrects the hypergastrinemia and decreases the basal acid secretory rate, heals any peptic ulcer and ameliorates any symptoms of gastroesophageal reflux [115]. Conversely, gastric ulcers are associated with *H. pylori*–induced pan- or corpus-predominant gastritis, resulting in multifocal atrophy of acid-secreting mucosa and reduced acid secretion. These ulcers usually arise at the junction of the antral and corpus mucosa, an area of intense inflammation [113]. Thus, the non-acidophilic nature of *H. pylori* (see section 1.2.1) explains how those with low acid secretory capacity are more susceptible to spread of infection through the corpus mucosa and to gastric ulceration. With their somewhat common pathobiology, gastric ulcer disease precedes the development of gastric cancer [93,116,117]. Gastric and duodenal ulcers have marked differences in their basis, placing them on opposite ends of disease spectrum. *H. pylori*-induced duodenal ulcer conveys a lower risk of developing a gastric cancer [117]. But, what makes it possible for *H. pylori* to be involved in both ends of disease spectrum? Although the mechanisms are unclear, the infecting strain itself may play a crucial role on the diverging point of this disease spectrum [16,93]. Moreover, the similarity between the phenotype of gastric ulcer and gastric cancer raises questions about the carcinogenic potential of the associated *H. pylori* strains [93]. Certainly the etiology for *H. pylori*-associated peptic ulcer in adults depends on the complex interplay of gastritis phenotype and of progressive physiological gastro-duodenal alterations through childhood until adulthood, a result of environmental factors, bacterial virulence factors and host genetic background.

Despite epidemiological evidence that infection during childhood is seldom associated with peptic ulceration or gastric atrophy, the mechanisms underlying differences in histopathology and clinical expression of *H. pylori* infection when compared to the adult, are still poorly identified. Theoretically, such differences might be explained by qualitative and/or quantitative differences in induced immune response, possibly age-related. Indeed, adults exhibit a predominantly neutrophil infiltrate, whereas *H. pylori*-associated gastritis in children is usually mild and superficial with a predominantly mononuclear infiltrate, a paucity of neutrophils and a higher degree of lymphoid follicular hyperplasia [118]. Therefore, different immunopathology and different patterns of cytokine expression would be anticipated for children when compared to adults [18]. There may be differences in adaptive component of gastric mucosa immune response in children compared to the adult host; a clear Th1 response has not always been demonstrated for young patients. The lower gastritis scores in children may also be a reflection of such a skewed Th1/Th2 balance, which may result in their lower risk for developing ulcer disease [18, 19]. These findings could indicate that the host humoral and cellular responses differ depending on the age at which the gastric infection is first acquired and might explain the varying rates of disease outcomes that are evident in different parts of the world. Nevertheless, higher anti-*H. pylori* IgG antibody titres occur in paediatric patients with duodenal ulcer compared to those without ulceration, suggesting that local humoral immune responses contribute to the development of peptic ulceration in these young patients [102,119,120]. This is not surprising, given the fact that the more severe inflammation, the greater the chance of ulcer formation [121] with increased IgG production leading to mucosal damage similar to an Arthus reaction [2].

1.3.3. Endoscopic features

Endoscopy is the only method to accurately diagnose peptic ulceration in children [87,122]. A nodular mucosa in the gastric antrum or duodenal bulb and/or gastric or duodenal erosions or ulcerations are specific (but not sensitive) features, suggesting active *H. pylori* infection. For those with suspected infection, biopsies should be obtained for histopathology, as well as complementary tests for detection of *H. pylori* including rapid urease test, histopathology with Giemsa stain and, if available, culture. The rationale for the recommendation to perform more than one diagnostic test is based on their sensitivity results in children, which range from 66% to 100% for histology and from 75% to 100% for rapid urease tests [91]. In all paediatric age groups, for patients receiving therapy with a proton pump inhibitor, biopsies should be performed on the body and cardia (and, possibly, transition zones) of the stomach as well as from the antrum to reduce the chances of false-negative results. Follow-up endoscopy is rarely necessary, except in the setting of peptic ulceration associated with complications (such as haemorrhage or perforation).

1.3.4. Host susceptibility

The multifactorial nature of peptic ulcer disease reflects its dependence on the patients' genetic susceptibility and habits (alcohol and/or non-steroid anti-inflammatory drug consumption, diet, smoking and stress) [20]. Paediatric peptic ulcer disease is significantly more frequent in boys than in girls (63.6% *versus* 36.4%, $p<0.025$) [32]. Although female hormones may have a protective role against developing peptic ulcerations [123], the true nature of this susceptibility of the male gender remains unclear.

Mucins, glycoproteins secreted by the gastric mucosa, form a gel layer that is essential to maintain a stable neutral pH adjacent to epithelium. This mucus barrier affords protection from attack by acid-pepsin and other luminal noxious agents [124]. *H. pylori* has a complex relationship with different gastric mucins' subtypes. Infected children for example have a decreased mucin in their gastric mucosa presumably weakening this important defense barrier [125]. The highly diverse carbohydrate structure of the gastric mucins, functioning as binding sites for *H. pylori*, should also play a role in the outcome of infection, with genetic and epigenetic changes in the mucin molecules influencing the susceptibility of the patient for *H. pylori*-associated peptic ulcer disease. Recently, it was shown that *H. pylori*-infected children presented a normal pattern of expression and glycosylation of mucin 5AC (MUC5AC) in the surface mucous cells, and MUC6 in the gland mucous cells, contrasting with the aberrant expression of MUC6 and MUC2 found in infected adults. Additionally, it was shown that the pattern of Lewis blood group antigens in the surface epithelium of children was significantly correlated with *H. pylori* load, however no correlation with gastritis, nodularity, and gastric or duodenal ulcer was found [17].

In children and teenagers, as in adults, the severity of antral inflammation strongly correlates with the risk of duodenal ulcer disease. Among the host factors, polymorphisms in cytokines encoding genes, or in their promoters, that affect cytokine transcription, are good risk candidates. Indeed, polymorphisms in the IL-1 gene cluster play an important role in modulating the risk for *H. pylori*-induced hypochlorhydria and, thus, for gastric ulceration and cancer. The

IL-1 cluster, located on chromosome 2q12-22 region, includes the genes *IL-1A, IL-1B* and *IL-1RN* that code for the proinflammatory cytokines IL-1α, IL-1β and their endogenous receptor antagonist IL-1RA, respectively. The less common alleles of *IL-1B, i.e., IL-1B-31C* and *IL-1B-511T* (representing, respectively, T-C and C-T transitions at positions 31 and 511 of the *IL-1B* promoter) are associated with a higher risk of hypochlorhydria [116]. This association can be explained considering that such polymorphisms lead to increased IL-1β expression/ secretion that, upon *H. pylori*-infection, amplifies the host inflammatory response. Also the less common allele of IL-1RA, *i.e.*, the IL-1RN*2 (representing one of the five known 86 base pair tandem repeat polymorphisms in intron 2) is associated with a higher risk of gastric cancer in adults [116]. The risk is potentiated when in association with infection by *cagA*/*vacA*-positive *H. pylori* strains, highlighting the interplay between host and bacterial factors that seems to be involved in the development of gastric pathology [126]. Children presenting the IL1RN*2 allele and infected by *cagA*-positive *H. pylori* strains are at higher risk of duodenal ulceration, emphasizing differences in the physiopathology of the disease between adult and paediatric patients [124]. Also at higher risk of developing duodenal ulcer are children presenting the transition G-A at position 238 of the TNF-α coding gene when infected by *iceA1*-positive *H. pylori* strains [127].

Other putative host risk factors for *H. pylori*-severe gastroduodenal diseases are the polymorphisms in the genes coding for Toll-like receptors (TLRs) that might influence the innate and adaptive immune response to the infection. Indeed, the presence of the TLR4 allele in combination with infection by *cagA*-positive strains, leads to increased gastric levels of IL-8 and IL-10 [128].

1.4. Molecular profile of ulcerogenic paediatric *H. pylori* strains

The co-evolution between *H. pylori* and the modern humans has determined the extremely high diversity of the bacterium in both its genetic background and virulence. Thus, it is likely that bacterial determinants may influence the clinical outcome, an association that is well established for *cagA, vacA* and *babA* genes (see sections 1.2.2 and 1.2.3 of this chapter). Nevertheless, this topic is far from being fully clarified, and the identification of other factors responsible for the enhanced virulence of the bacteria leading to the development of more severe diseases remains pertinent. For that purpose, the study of *H. pylori* strains isolated in specific clinical situations, such as the paediatric peptic ulcer disease, can be useful. Indeed, *H. pylori* paediatric infection may be regarded as a privileged natural study model of the interaction of this bacterium with human host, as the child is usually not exposed to injurious factors as is the adult and represents a different stage of *H. pylori* infection in a immunologically maturing host. Comparative genomic studies of the rare paediatric ulcerogenic *H. pylori* strains and of the non-ulcerogenic strains show a distinctive genotype virulence pattern, suggesting a potential pathogenic role for new markers [9-15]. Two putative virulence determinants are associated with peptic ulceration, mostly duodenal ulcer, in children and with other *H. pylori*-virulence factors: *jhp0562,* involved in lipopolysaccharide biosynthesis and in the regulation of Lewis antigen expression [13]; and *homB*, a putative outer membrane protein, involved in bacterial adherence [9,11,12,14,15]. HomB contributes to the proinflammatory characteristics of *H. pylori*. Strains that are also positive for both *homB* and *jhp562* are related to a higher risk of paediatric peptic ulcer disease. Thus, it is likely that these new markers acting together with the well-established virulence markers will promote a more severe antral inflammation, a phenomenon strongly associated with duodenal ulceration.

Other pathogenic genes interact synergistically to induce peptic ulcer in young patients. There is no gene or protein that acts alone to establish the virulence of *H. pylori* [74]. Accordingly, we investigated further virulence-associated genes by comparing the proteome of a group of genetically/epidemiologically-unlinked *H. pylori* strains, all isolated from Portuguese children, half suffering with peptic ulcer disease, and the other presenting only active gastritis [16]. Despite the typical proteome profile of all the *H. pylori* strains grown under the same laboratorial conditions [129], the ulcerogenic paediatric *H. pylori* strains presented differences suggestive of higher motility, better antioxidant defences and a metabolism favouring the biosynthesis of aromatic amino acids. As already mentioned in this chapter (see section 1.2.1 of this chapter) motility is a long known virulence-related trait [46], with lower-motility associated reduced inflammation levels [47] and with non-motile strains unable to establish a robust infection [42,45,46]. Moreover, it was more recently shown that higher motility enhances *H. pylori* density and inflammatory response in dyspeptic patients [130].

The differences in the abundance of antioxidant proteins observed between paediatric ulcerogenic and non-ulcerogenic strains may be important in conferring resistance to inflammation; the enzymes involved in key steps in the metabolism of glucose, amino acids and urea may be advantageous to respond to fluctuations of nutrients [16].

Additionally, by comparing the duodenal ulcer-associated paediatric strains with the one studied strain associated with gastric ulcer, we observed differences on the abundance of proteins associated with acid resistance and motility. These suggest that the former are better prepared to survive to the abnormal low levels of pH observed in duodenal ulceration, in contrast to the gastric ulcer strain which is a better swimmer, supporting the proximal spread of infection characteristic of this disease [16]. Overall, our data supports the idea that the infecting strain may be determinant in the divergence between duodenal and gastric ulcer [93].

2. Conclusions

The prevalence of *H. pylori* infection remains high worldwide despite a progressive decline over time, attributed to improved overall living conditions and hygiene. Although often asymptomatic, most infected patients suffer from persistent non-ulcer dyspepsia that, usually later in adulthood, may further progress to more severe conditions. The most common severe complication *H. pylori* is duodenal ulcer, affecting 10 to 15% of the infected adults. Although less frequent, 2 to 5% of the infected adults with non-ulcer dyspepsia progress to gastric ulceration and some ultimately to gastric cancer. These two forms of peptic ulcer-related (organic) dyspepsia differ in prevalence and physiopathology; those suffering with duodenal ulcer are at low risk of developing a gastric ulcer/gastric cancer. The onset of peptic ulcers in childhood is a rare event that may occur shortly after infection, suggesting more virulent *H.*

pylori strains and more susceptible young patients. *H. pylori*-associated paediatric peptic ulcer disease is, therefore, a privileged natural study model to search for ulcerogenic-specific bacterial biomarkers and implicated molecular mechanisms, a required step to better address this important public health problem. This includes enhanced virulence of the paediatric ulcerogenic *H. pylori* strains that also may have a natural ability to better adapt to the hostility of their niche.

Acknowledgements

This work was supported by BNP Paribas patronage and a research Grant from the Sociedade Portuguesa de Gastrenterologia.

Author details

Mónica Roxo-Rosa[1], Mónica Oleastro[2] and Ana Isabel Lopes[3]

*Address all correspondence to: roxorosa@hotmail.com

1 Center for Biodiversity, Functional & Integrative Genomics, Faculty of Sciences, University of Lisbon, Lisbon, Portugal and Department of Genetics, National Institute of Health Dr. Ricardo Jorge, Lisbon, Portugal

2 Department of Infectious Diseases, National Institute of Health Dr. Ricardo Jorge, Lisbon, Portugal

3 Gastroenterology Unit, Department of Paediatrics, University Hospital Santa Maria, Medical Faculty of Lisbon, Lisbon, Portugal

References

[1] Linz B, Balloux F, Moodley Y, Manica A, Liu H, Roumagnac P et al. An African origin for the intimate association between humans and Helicobacter pylori. Nature 2007; 445(7130):915-918.

[2] Blaser MJ. Helicobacters are indigenous to the human stomach: duodenal ulceration is due to changes in gastric microecology in the modern era. Gut 1998; 43(5):721-727.

[3] Konturek PC, Konturek SJ, Brzozowski T. Helicobacter pylori infection in gastric cancerogenesis. J Physiol Pharmacol 2009; 60(3):3-21.

[4] Pacifico L, Anania C, Osborn JF, Ferraro F, Chiesa C. Consequences of Helicobacter pylori infection in children. World J Gastroenterol 2010; 16(41):5181-5194.

[5] Oderda G, Shcherbakov P, Bontems P, Urruzuno P, Romano C, Gottrand F et al. Results from the pediatric European register for treatment of Helicobacter pylori (PERTH). Helicobacter 2007; 12(2):150-156.

[6] Oderda G, Mura S, Valori A, Brustia R. Idiopathic peptic ulcers in children. J Pediatr Gastroenterol Nutr 2009; 48(3):268-270.

[7] Tam YH, Lee KH, To KF, Chan KW, Cheung ST. Helicobacter pylori-positive versus Helicobacter pylori-negative idiopathic peptic ulcers in children with their long-term outcomes. J Pediatr Gastroenterol Nutr 2009; 48(3):299-305.

[8] Kalach N, Bontems P, Koletzko S, Mourad-Baars P, Shcherbakov P, Celinska-Cedro D et al. Frequency and risk factors of gastric and duodenal ulcers or erosions in children: a prospective 1-month European multicenter study. Eur J Gastroenterol Hepatol 2010; 22(10):1174-1181.

[9] Oleastro M, Cordeiro R, Ferrand J, Nunes B, Lehours P, Carvalho-Oliveira I et al. Evaluation of the clinical significance of homB, a novel candidate marker of Helicobacter pylori strains associated with peptic ulcer disease. J Infect Dis 2008; 198(9): 1379-1387.

[10] Lopes AI, Palha A, Monteiro L, Olcastro M, Pelerito A, Fernandes A. Helicobacter pylori genotypes in children from a population at high gastric cancer risk: no association with gastroduodenal histopathology. Am J Gastroenterol 2006; 101(9):2113-2122.

[11] Oleastro M, Monteiro L, Lehours P, Megraud F, Menard A. Identification of markers for Helicobacter pylori strains isolated from children with peptic ulcer disease by suppressive subtractive hybridization. Infect Immun 2006; 74(7):4064-4074.

[12] Oleastro M, Cordeiro R, Yamaoka Y, Queiroz D, Megraud F, Monteiro L et al. Disease association with two Helicobacter pylori duplicate outer membrane protein genes, homB and homA. Gut Pathog 2009; 1(1):12.

[13] Oleastro M, Santos A, Cordeiro R, Nunes B, Megraud F, Menard A. Clinical relevance and diversity of two homologous genes encoding glycosyltransferases in Helicobacter pylori. J Clin Microbiol 2010; 48(8):2885-2891.

[14] Oleastro M, Gerhard M, Lopes AI, Ramalho P, Cabral J, Sousa GA et al. Helicobacter pylori virulence genotypes in Portuguese children and adults with gastroduodenal pathology. Eur J Clin Microbiol Infect Dis 2003; 22(2):85-91.

[15] Oleastro M, Cordeiro R, Menard A, Yamaoka Y, Queiroz D, Megraud F et al. Allelic diversity and phylogeny of homB, a novel co-virulence marker of Helicobacter pylori. BMC Microbiol 2009; 9(1):248.

[16] Vitoriano I, Saraiva-Pava KD, Rocha-Goncalves A, Santos A, Lopes AI, Oleastro M et al. Ulcerogenic Helicobacter pylori strains isolated from children: a contribution to get insight into the virulence of the bacteria. PLoS ONE 2011; 6(10):e26265.

[17] Linden S, Semino-Mora C, Liu H, Rick J, Dubois A. Role of mucin Lewis status in resistance to Helicobacter pylori infection in pediatric patients. Helicobacter 2010; 15(4):251-258.

[18] Lopes AI, Quiding-Jarbrink M, Palha A, Ruivo J, Monteiro L, Oleastro M et al. Cytokine expression in pediatric Helicobacter pylori infection. Clin Diagn Lab Immunol 2005; 12(8):994-1002.

[19] Lopes AI, Victorino RM, Palha AM, Ruivo J, Fernandes A. Mucosal lymphocyte subsets and HLA-DR antigen expression in paediatric Helicobacter pylori-associated gastritis. Clin Exp Immunol 2006; 145(1):13-20.

[20] Salles N, Megraud F. Current management of Helicobacter pylori infections in the elderly. Expert Rev Anti Infect Ther 2007; 5(5):845-856.

[21] Rowland M, Daly L, Vaughan M, Higgins A, Bourke B, Drumm B. Age-specific incidence of Helicobacter pylori. Gastroenterology 2006; 130(1):65-72.

[22] Goodman KJ, O'rourke K, Day RS, Wang C, Nurgalieva Z, Phillips CV et al. Dynamics of Helicobacter pylori infection in a US-Mexico cohort during the first two years of life. Int J Epidemiol 2005; 34(6):1348-1355.

[23] Mitchell H, Megraud F. Epidemiology and diagnosis of Helicobacter pylori infection. Helicobacter 2002; 7 Suppl 1:8-16.

[24] Bardhan PK. Epidemiological features of Helicobacter pylori infection in developing countries. Clin Infect Dis 1997; 25(5):973-978.

[25] Kawakami E, Machado RS, Ogata SK, Langner M. Decrease in prevalence of Helicobacter pylori infection during a 10-year period in Brazilian children. Arq Gastroenterol 2008; 45(2):147-151.

[26] Elitsur Y, Dementieva Y, Rewalt M, Lawrence Z. Helicobacter pylori infection rate decreases in symptomatic children: a retrospective analysis of 13 years (1993-2005) from a gastroenterology clinic in West Virginia. J Clin Gastroenterol 2009; 43(2): 147-151.

[27] Azevedo NF, Huntington J, Goodman KJ. The epidemiology of Helicobacter pylori and public health implications. Helicobacter 2009; 14 Suppl 1:1-7.

[28] Oleastro M, Pelerito A, Nogueira P, Benoliel J, Santos A, Cabral J et al. Prevalence and incidence of Helicobacter pylori Infection in a healthy pediatric population in the Lisbon area. Helicobacter 2011; 16(5):363-372.

[29] Quina MG. Helicobacter pylori: the Portuguese scene. Grupo de Estudo Portugues do Helicobacter pylori (GEPHP). Eur J Cancer Prev 1994; 3 Suppl 2:65-67.

[30] Vitoriano I, Rocha-Goncalves A, Carvalho T, Oleastro M, Calado CR, Roxo-Rosa M. Antigenic Diversity Among Portuguese Clinical Isolates of Helicobacter pylori. Helicobacter 2011; 16(2):153-168.

[31] Lopes AI, Oleastro M, Palha A, Fernandes A, Monteiro L. Antibiotic-resistant Helicobacter pylori strains in Portuguese children. Pediatr Infect Dis J 2005; 24(5):404-409.

[32] Oleastro M, Cabral J, Ramalho PM, Lemos PS, Paixao E, Benoliel J et al. Primary antibiotic resistance of Helicobacter pylori strains isolated from Portuguese children: a prospective multicentre study over a 10 year period. J Antimicrob Chemother 2011; 66(10):2308-2311.

[33] Vale FF, Roxo-Rosa M, Oleastro M. *Helicobacter pylori* resistance to antibiotics. In: A.Méndez-Vilas. (ed.) Science against microbial pathogens: communicating current research and technological advances. 2011. p745-756.

[34] Megraud F, Coenen S, Versporten A, Kist M, Lopez-Brea M, Hirschl AM et al. Helicobacter pylori resistance to antibiotics in Europe and its relationship to antibiotic consumption. Gut 2013; 62(1):34-42.

[35] De F, V, Giorgio F, Hassan C, Manes G, Vannella L, Panella C et al. Worldwide H. pylori antibiotic resistance: a systematic review. J Gastrointestin Liver Dis 2010; 19(4): 409-414.

[36] Yamade M, Sugimoto M, Uotani T, Nishino M, Kodaira C, Furuta T. Resistance of Helicobacter pylori to quinolones and clarithromycin assessed by genetic testing in Japan. J Gastroenterol Hepatol 2011; 26(9):1457-1461.

[37] Koletzko S, Richy F, Bontems P, Crone J, Kalach N, Monteiro ML et al. Prospective multicentre study on antibiotic resistance of Helicobacter pylori strains obtained from children living in Europe. Gut 2006; 55(12):1711-1716.

[38] Agudo S, Alarcon T, Cibrelus L, Urruzuno P, Martinez MJ, Lopez-Brea M. [High percentage of clarithromycin and metronidazole resistance in Helicobacter pylori clinical isolates obtained from Spanish children]. Rev Esp Quimioter 2009; 22(2):88-92.

[39] Stingl K, De Reuse H. Staying alive overdosed: how does Helicobacter pylori control urease activity? Int J Med Microbiol 2005; 295(5):307-315.

[40] Benoit SL, Maier RJ. Mua (HP0868) is a nickel-binding protein that modulates urease activity in Helicobacter pylori. MBio 2011; 2(2):e00039-11.

[41] Schreiber S, Konradt M, Groll C, Scheid P, Hanauer G, Werling HO et al. The spatial orientation of Helicobacter pylori in the gastric mucus. Proc Natl Acad Sci U S A 2004; 101(14):5024-5029.

[42] Ottemann KM, Lowenthal AC. Helicobacter pylori uses motility for initial colonization and to attain robust infection. Infect Immun 2002; 70(4):1984-1990.

[43] Hazell SL, Lee A, Brady L, Hennessy W. Campylobacter pyloridis and gastritis: association with intercellular spaces and adaptation to an environment of mucus as im-

portant factors in colonization of the gastric epithelium. J Infect Dis 1986; 153(4): 658-663.

[44] Sycuro LK, Pincus Z, Gutierrez KD, Biboy J, Stern CA, Vollmer W et al. Peptidoglycan crosslinking relaxation promotes Helicobacter pylori's helical shape and stomach colonization. Cell 2010; 141(5):822-833.

[45] Josenhans C, Labigne A, Suerbaum S. Comparative ultrastructural and functional studies of Helicobacter pylori and Helicobacter mustelae flagellin mutants: both flagellin subunits, FlaA and FlaB, are necessary for full motility in Helicobacter species. J Bacteriol 1995; 177(11):3010-3020.

[46] Eaton KA, Suerbaum S, Josenhans C, Krakowka S. Colonization of gnotobiotic piglets by Helicobacter pylori deficient in two flagellin genes. Infect Immun 1996; 64(7): 2445-2448.

[47] Watanabe S, Takagi A, Tada U, Kabir AM, Koga Y, Kamiya S et al. Cytotoxicity and motility of Helicobacter pylori. PG - S169-71 AB - To clarify the relationship between interleukin-8 (IL-8) production and virulent factors, we examined the motility and cytotoxicity of H. pylori, suggested to be a major cause of chronic gastritis and peptic ulcers. Our results demonstrated that among cytotoxic strains of H. pylori, high-motility strains induced more IL-8 than low-motility strains. There was no correlation between cytotoxicity and motility of H. pylori. Four restriction fragment length polymorphism (RFLP) patterns were observed in the flaA PCR products. There was no correlation between flaA RFLP and motility. In conclusion, our findings suggest that both cytotoxicity and motility are virulent factors in the pathogenesis of gastric mucosal injury. J Clin Gastroenterol 1997; 25 Suppl 1.

[48] Dubois A, Boren T. Helicobacter pylori is invasive and it may be a facultative intracellular organism. Cell Microbiol 2007; 9(5):1108-1116.

[49] Ilver D, Arnqvist A, Ogren J, Frick IM, Kersulyte D, Incecik ET et al. Helicobacter pylori adhesin binding fucosylated histo-blood group antigens revealed by retagging. Science 1998; 279(5349):373-377.

[50] Ohno T, Vallstrom A, Rugge M, Ota H, Graham DY, Arnqvist A et al. Effects of blood group antigen-binding adhesin expression during Helicobacter pylori infection of Mongolian gerbils. J Infect Dis 2011; 203(5):726-735.

[51] Fujimoto S, Olaniyi OO, Arnqvist A, Wu JY, Odenbreit S, Haas R et al. Helicobacter pylori BabA expression, gastric mucosal injury, and clinical outcome. Clin Gastroenterol Hepatol 2007; 5(1):49-58.

[52] Mahdavi J, Sonden B, Hurtig M, Olfat FO, Forsberg L, Roche N et al. Helicobacter pylori SabA adhesin in persistent infection and chronic inflammation. Science 2002; 297(5581):573-578.

[53] Sakamoto S, Watanabe T, Tokumaru T, Takagi H, Nakazato H, Lloyd KO. Expression of Lewisa, Lewisb, Lewisx, Lewisy, siayl-Lewisa, and sialyl-Lewisx blood group anti-

gens in human gastric carcinoma and in normal gastric tissue. Cancer Res 1989; 49(3): 745-752.

[54] Ota H, Nakayama J, Momose M, Hayama M, Akamatsu T, Katsuyama T et al. Helicobacter pylori infection produces reversible glycosylation changes to gastric mucins. Virchows Arch 1998; 433(5):419-426.

[55] Aspholm M, Olfat FO, Norden J, Sonden B, Lundberg C, Sjostrom R et al. SabA is the H. pylori hemagglutinin and is polymorphic in binding to sialylated glycans. PLoS Pathog 2006; 2(10):e110.

[56] Unemo M, Aspholm-Hurtig M, Ilver D, Bergstrom J, Boren T, Danielsson D et al. The sialic acid binding SabA adhesin of Helicobacter pylori is essential for nonopsonic activation of human neutrophils. J Biol Chem 2005; 280(15):15390-15397.

[57] Yamaoka Y, Kwon DH, Graham DY. A M(r) 34,000 proinflammatory outer membrane protein (oipA) of Helicobacter pylori. Proc Natl Acad Sci U S A 2000; 97(13): 7533-7538.

[58] Yamaoka Y, Ojo O, Fujimoto S, Odenbreit S, Haas R, Gutierrez O et al. Helicobacter pylori outer membrane proteins and gastroduodenal disease. Gut 2006; 55(6):775-781.

[59] Franco AT, Johnston E, Krishna U, Yamaoka Y, Israel DA, Nagy TA et al. Regulation of gastric carcinogenesis by Helicobacter pylori virulence factors. Cancer Res 2008; 68(2):379-387.

[60] Censini S, Lange C, Xiang Z, Crabtree JE, Ghiara P, Borodovsky M et al. cag, a pathogenicity island of Helicobacter pylori, encodes type I-specific and disease-associated virulence factors. Proc Natl Acad Sci U S A 1996; 93(25):14648-14653.

[61] Covacci A, Rappuoli R. Tyrosine-phosphorylated bacterial proteins: Trojan horses for the host cell. J Exp Med 2000; 191(4):587-592.

[62] Parker H, Keenan JI. Composition and function of Helicobacter pylori outer membrane vesicles. Microbes Infect 2012; 14(1):9-16.

[63] Backert S, Tegtmeyer N, Selbach M. The versatility of Helicobacter pylori CagA effector protein functions: The master key hypothesis. Helicobacter 2010; 15(3):163-176.

[64] Blaser MJ, Perez-Perez GI, Kleanthous H, Cover TL, Peek RM, Chyou PH et al. Infection with Helicobacter pylori strains possessing cagA is associated with an increased risk of developing adenocarcinoma of the stomach. Cancer Res 1995; 55(10): 2111-2115.

[65] Covacci A, Censini S, Bugnoli M, Petracca R, Burroni D, Macchia G et al. Molecular characterization of the 128-kDa immunodominant antigen of Helicobacter pylori associated with cytotoxicity and duodenal ulcer. Proc Natl Acad Sci U S A 1993; 90(12): 5791-5795.

[66] Ohnishi N, Yuasa H, Tanaka S, Sawa H, Miura M, Matsui A et al. Transgenic expression of Helicobacter pylori CagA induces gastrointestinal and hematopoietic neoplasms in mouse. Proc Natl Acad Sci U S A 2008; 105(3):1003-1008.

[67] Ferreira RM, Machado JC, Figueiredo C. Variation in Helicobacter pylori cagA promoter region is associated with CagA expression. Helicobacter 2012; 17(S1):W1.5.

[68] Palframan SL, Kwok T, Gabriel K. Vacuolating cytotoxin A (VacA), a key toxin for Helicobacter pylori pathogenesis. Front Cell Infect Microbiol 2012; 2:92.

[69] Chambers MG, Pyburn TM, Gonzalez-Rivera C, Collier SE, Eli I, Yip CK et al. Structural Analysis of the Oligomeric States of Helicobacter pylori VacA Toxin. J Mol Biol 2012.

[70] Gangwer KA, Mushrush DJ, Stauff DL, Spiller B, McClain MS, Cover TL et al. Crystal structure of the Helicobacter pylori vacuolating toxin p55 domain. Proc Natl Acad Sci U S A 2007; 104(41):16293-16298.

[71] Boquet P, Ricci V, Galmiche A, Gauthier NC. Gastric cell apoptosis and H. pylori: has the main function of VacA finally been identified? Trends Microbiol 2003; 11(9): 410-413.

[72] Cover TL, Blanke SR. Helicobacter pylori VacA, a paradigm for toxin multifunctionality. Nat Rev Microbiol 2005; 3(4):320-332.

[73] Rieder G, Fischer W, Haas R. Interaction of Helicobacter pylori with host cells: function of secreted and translocated molecules. Curr Opin Microbiol 2005; 8(1):67-73.

[74] Yamaoka Y. Pathogenesis of Helicobacter pylori-Related Gastroduodenal Diseases from Molecular Epidemiological Studies. Gastroenterol Res Pract 2012; 2012:371503.

[75] Tham KT, Peek RM, Jr., Atherton JC, Cover TL, Perez-Perez GI, Shyr Y et al. Helicobacter pylori genotypes, host factors, and gastric mucosal histopathology in peptic ulcer disease. Hum Pathol 2001; 32(3):264-273.

[76] Israel DA, Peek RM. Surreptitious manipulation of the human host by Helicobacter pylori. Gut Microbes 2010; 1(2):119-127.

[77] Moran AP, Hynes SO, Heneghan MA. Mimicry of blood group antigen A by Helicobacter mustelae and H. pylori. Gastroenterology 1999; 116(2):504-505.

[78] Jonsson K, Guo BP, Monstein HJ, Mekalanos JJ, Kronvall G. Molecular cloning and characterization of two Helicobacter pylori genes coding for plasminogen-binding proteins. Proc Natl Acad Sci U S A 2004; 101(7):1852-1857.

[79] Axsen WS, Styer CM, Solnick JV. Inhibition of heat shock protein expression by Helicobacter pylori. Microb Pathog 2009; 47(4):231-236.

[80] Solnick JV, Hansen LM, Salama NR, Boonjakuakul JK, Syvanen M. Modification of Helicobacter pylori outer membrane protein expression during experimental infection of rhesus macaques. Proc Natl Acad Sci U S A 2004; 101(7):2106-2111.

[81] Carvalho MA, Machado NC, Ortolan EV, Rodrigues MA. Upper gastrointestinal histopathological findings in children and adolescents with nonulcer dyspepsia with Helicobacter pylori infection. J Pediatr Gastroenterol Nutr 2012; 55(5):523-529.

[82] Sood MR, Joshi S, Akobeng AK, Mitchell J, Thomas AG. Growth in children with Helicobacter pylori infection and dyspepsia. Arch Dis Child 2005; 90(10):1025-1028.

[83] Yang YJ, Sheu BS, Lee SC, Yang HB, Wu JJ. Children of Helicobacter pylori-infected dyspeptic mothers are predisposed to H. pylori acquisition with subsequent iron deficiency and growth retardation. Helicobacter 2005; 10(3):249-255.

[84] Farrell S, Milliken I, Murphy JL, Wootton SA, McCallion WA. Nonulcer dyspepsia and Helicobacter pylori eradication in children. J Pediatr Surg 2005; 40(10):1547-1550.

[85] Kalach N, Mention K, Guimber D, Michaud L, Spyckerelle C, Gottrand F. Helicobacter pylori infection is not associated with specific symptoms in nonulcer-dyspeptic children. Pediatrics 2005; 115(1):17-21.

[86] Bourke B, Ceponis P, Chiba N, Czinn S, Ferraro R, Fischbach L et al. Canadian Helicobacter Study Group Consensus Conference: Update on the approach to Helicobacter pylori infection in children and adolescents--an evidence-based evaluation. Can J Gastroenterol 2005; 19(7):399-408.

[87] Malfertheiner P, Megraud F, O'Morain C, Bazzoli F, El Omar E, Graham D et al. Current concepts in the management of Helicobacter pylori infection: the Maastricht III Consensus Report. Gut 2007; 56(6):772-781.

[88] Tindberg Y, Nyren O, Blennow M, Granstrom M. Helicobacter pylori infection and abdominal symptoms among Swedish school children. J Pediatr Gastroenterol Nutr 2005; 41(1):33-38.

[89] Bode G, Brenner H, Adler G, Rothenbacher D. Recurrent abdominal pain in children: evidence from a population-based study that social and familial factors play a major role but not Helicobacter pylori infection. J Psychosom Res 2003; 54(5):417-421.

[90] Perez ME, Youssef NN. Dyspepsia in childhood and adolescence: insights and treatment considerations. Curr Gastroenterol Rep 2007; 9(6):447-455.

[91] Koletzko S, Jones NL, Goodman KJ, Gold B, Rowland M, Cadranel S et al. Evidence-based guidelines from ESPGHAN and NASPGHAN for Helicobacter pylori infection in children. J Pediatr Gastroenterol Nutr 2011; 53(2):230-243.

[92] Drumm B, Rhoads JM, Stringer DA, Sherman PM, Ellis LE, Durie PR. Peptic ulcer disease in children: etiology, clinical findings, and clinical course. Pediatrics 1988; 82(3 Pt 2):410-414.

[93] Ubukata H, Nagata H, Tabuchi T, Konishi S, Kasuga T, Tabuchi T. Why is the coexistence of gastric cancer and duodenal ulcer rare? Examination of factors related to both gastric cancer and duodenal ulcer. Gastric Cancer 2011; 14(1):4-12.

[94] Arents NL, Thijs JC, van Zwet AA, Kleibeuker JH. Does the declining prevalence of Helicobacter pylori unmask patients with idiopathic peptic ulcer disease? Trends over an 8 year period. Eur J Gastroenterol Hepatol 2004; 16(8):779-783.

[95] Vakil N. Dyspepsia, peptic ulcer, and H. pylori: a remembrance of things past. Am J Gastroenterol 2010; 105(3):572-574.

[96] Sherman P, Czinn S, Drumm B, Gottrand F, Kawakami E, Madrazo A et al. Helicobacter pylori infection in children and adolescents: Working Group Report of the First World Congress of Pediatric Gastroenterology, Hepatology, and Nutrition. J Pediatr Gastroenterol Nutr 2002; 35 Suppl 2:S128-S133.

[97] Bourke B, Sherman P, Drumm B. Peptic ulcer disease: what is the role for Helicobacter pylori? Semin Gastrointest Dis 1994; 5(1):24-31.

[98] Kneepkens C.M.F. Peptic ulcer disease in childhood. Acta Endosc 1994; 24:169-181.

[99] Oderda G, Ansaldi N. Peptic ulcers in childhood. Lancet 1988; 1(8580):302-303.

[100] Egbaria R, Levine A, Tamir A, Shaoul R. Peptic ulcers and erosions are common in Israeli children undergoing upper endoscopy. Helicobacter 2008; 13(1):62-68.

[101] Kato S, Nishino Y, Ozawa K, Konno M, Maisawa S, Toyoda S et al. The prevalence of Helicobacter pylori in Japanese children with gastritis or peptic ulcer disease. J Gastroenterol 2004; 39(8):734-738.

[102] Nijevitch AA, Sataev VU, Vakhitov VA, Loguinovskaya VV, Kotsenko TM. Childhood peptic ulcer in the Ural area of Russia: clinical status and Helicobacter pylori-associated immune response. J Pediatr Gastroenterol Nutr 2001; 33(5):558-564.

[103] Walsh JH, Peterson WL. The treatment of Helicobacter pylori infection in the management of peptic ulcer disease. N Engl J Med 1995; 333(15):984-991.

[104] Macarthur C, Saunders N, Feldman W. Helicobacter pylori, gastroduodenal disease, and recurrent abdominal pain in children. JAMA 1995; 273(9):729-734.

[105] Brown K, Lundborg P, Levinson J, Yang H. Incidence of peptic ulcer bleeding in the US pediatric population. J Pediatr Gastroenterol Nutr 2012; 54(6):733-736.

[106] Khurana R, Fischbach L, Chiba N, VAN Zanten SV, Sherman PM, George BA et al. Meta-analysis: Helicobacter pylori eradication treatment efficacy in children. Aliment Pharmacol Ther 2007; 25(5):523-536.

[107] Ford AC, Delaney BC, Forman D, Moayyedi P. Eradication therapy for peptic ulcer disease in Helicobacter pylori positive patients. Cochrane Database Syst Rev 2006; (2):CD003840.

[108] Kato S, Sherman PM. What is new related to Helicobacter pylori infection in children and teenagers? Arch Pediatr Adolesc Med 2005; 159(5):415-421.

[109] Goggin N, Rowland M, Imrie C, Walsh D, Clyne M, Drumm B. Effect of Helicobacter pylori eradication on the natural history of duodenal ulcer disease. Arch Dis Child 1998; 79(6):502-505.

[110] Chiesa C, Pacifico L, Anania C, Poggiogalle E, Chiarelli F, Osborn JF. Helicobacter pylori therapy in children: overview and challenges. Int J Immunopathol Pharmacol 2010; 23(2):405-416.

[111] Sherman P, Hassall E, Hunt RH, Fallone CA, Veldhuyzen VZ, Thomson AB. Canadian Helicobacter Study Group Consensus Conference on the Approach to Helicobacter pylori Infection in Children and Adolescents. Can J Gastroenterol 1999; 13(7): 553-559.

[112] Huang FC, Chang MH, Hsu HY, Lee PI, Shun CT. Long-term follow-up of duodenal ulcer in children before and after eradication of Helicobacter pylori. J Pediatr Gastroenterol Nutr 1999; 28(1):76-80.

[113] Tytgat GN. Etiopathogenetic principles and peptic ulcer disease classification. Dig Dis 2011; 29(5):454-458.

[114] Atherton JC, Blaser MJ. Coadaptation of Helicobacter pylori and humans: ancient history, modern implications. J Clin Invest 2009; 119(9):2475-2487.

[115] Osefo N, Ito T, Jensen RT. Gastric acid hypersecretory states: recent insights and advances. Curr Gastroenterol Rep 2009; 11(6):433-441.

[116] El Omar EM, Carrington M, Chow WH, McColl KE, Bream JH, Young HA et al. Interleukin-1 polymorphisms associated with increased risk of gastric cancer. Nature 2000; 404(6776):398-402.

[117] Hansson LE, Nyren O, Hsing AW, Bergstrom R, Josefsson S, Chow WH et al. The risk of stomach cancer in patients with gastric or duodenal ulcer disease. N Engl J Med 1996; 335(4):242-249.

[118] Whitney AE, Guarner J, Hutwagner L, Gold BD. Helicobacter pylori gastritis in children and adults: comparative histopathologic study. Ann Diagn Pathol 2000; 4(5): 279-285.

[119] de Oliveira AM, Rocha GA, Queiroz DM, Mendes EN, de Carvalho AS, Ferrari TC et al. Evaluation of enzyme-linked immunosorbent assay for the diagnosis of Helicobacter pylori infection in children from different age groups with and without duodenal ulcer. J Pediatr Gastroenterol Nutr 1999; 28(2):157-161.

[120] Oderda G, Vaira D, Holton J, Ainley C, Altare F, Boero M et al. Helicobacter pylori in children with peptic ulcer and their families. Dig Dis Sci 1991; 36(5):572-576.

[121] Lee A. Future research in peptic ulcer disease. Scand J Gastroenterol Suppl 1994; 205:51-58.

[122] Drumm B, Day AS, Gold B, Gottrand F, Kato S, Kawakami E et al. Helicobacter pylori and peptic ulcer: Working Group Report of the second World Congress of Pediatric Gastroenterology, Hepatology, and Nutrition. J Pediatr Gastroenterol Nutr 2004; 39 Suppl 2:S626-S631.

[123] Schubert TT, Bologna SD, Nensey Y, Schubert AB, Mascha EJ, Ma CK. Ulcer risk factors: interactions between Helicobacter pylori infection, nonsteroidal use, and age. Am J Med 1993; 94(4):413-418.

[124] Niv Y, Boltin D. Secreted and membrane-bound mucins and idiopathic peptic ulcer disease. Digestion 2012; 86(3):258-263.

[125] Yamashiro Y, Oguchi S, Otsuka Y, Nagata S, Shioya T, Shimizu T. Helicobacter pylori colonization in children with gastritis and peptic ulcer. I. The colonization rate and effects of colonization on mucin content and mucosal inflammation in the antrum. Acta Paediatr Jpn 1994; 36(2):167-170.

[126] Rad R, Prinz C, Neu B, Neuhofer M, Zeitner M, Voland P et al. Synergistic effect of Helicobacter pylori virulence factors and interleukin-1 polymorphisms for the development of severe histological changes in the gastric mucosa. J Infect Dis 2003; 188(2): 272-281.

[127] Wilschanski M, Schlesinger Y, Faber J, Rudensky B, Ohnona FS, Freier S et al. Combination of Helicobacter pylori strain and tumor necrosis factor-alpha polymorphism of the host increases the risk of peptic ulcer disease in children. J Pediatr Gastroenterol Nutr 2007; 45(2):199-203.

[128] Moura SB, Almeida LR, Guerra JB, Rocha GA, Camargos Rocha AM, Melo FF et al. Toll-like receptor (TLR2, TLR4 and TLR5) gene polymorphisms and Helicobacter pylori infection in children with and without duodenal ulcer. Microbes Infect 2008; 10(14-15):1477-1483.

[129] Jungblut PR, Pleissner KP, Stein R, Butnner S, Knipper J. http://web.mpiib-berlin.mpg.de/cgi-bin/pdbs/2d-page/extern/index.cgi. Proteome 2D-PAGE Database - Home

[130] Kao CY, Sheu BS, Sheu SM, Yang HB, Chang WL, Cheng HC et al. Higher motility enhances bacterial density and inflammatory response in dyspeptic patients infected with Helicobacter pylori. Helicobacter 2012; 17(6):411-416.

Chapter 6

Diet in the Etiology and Management of Functional Dyspepsia

Jan Pen

Additional information is available at the end of the chapter

http://dx.doi.org/10.5772/57138

1. Introduction

Functional dyspepsia (FD) is a highly prevalent disorder, characterized by persistent or recurrent pain or discomfort centered in the upper abdomen without evidence of organic disease that might explain the symptoms [1]. Epidemiologic surveys suggest that 15 – 20 % of the general population in Western countries experience dyspepsia over the course of one year.

The options for managing functional dyspepsia are limited and far from ideal [2]. Limited information concerning the underlying pathophysiologic mechanisms has hampered the development of effective management strategies and specific therapeutic agents.

Several factors have been proposed to play a role in functional dyspepsia: delayed gastric emptying, *Helicobacter pylori* infection, hypersensitivity to gastric distention, impaired gastric accommodation to a meal, altered duodenal sensitivity to lipids or acids, abnormal duodeno-jejunal motility, and central nervous dysfunction. None of these abnormalities are able to completely account for the dyspepsia symptom complex [3].

Abnormal gastric motility and visceral hypersensitivity are generally thought to be directly linked to FD symptoms. Other factors that directly affect physiologic function include lifestyle, diet and genetics. [4,5]

The purpose of this chapter is to provide more specific dietary patterns and avoidances of certain food items in managing functional dyspepsia

2. Physiology of human feeding

The gastrointestinal tract processes ingested food via a complex series of actions in specific organs.

The esophagus propels food into the stomach though a relaxed lower esophageal sphincter that subsequently contracts to prevent gastroesophageal reflux. The functions of the proximal and distal stomach differ remarkably. Initially, the proximal stomach relaxes, providing a reservoir function. The distal stomach regulates the gastric emptying of solids by grinding and sieving the contents until the particles are small enough to pass the pylorus. The small intestine also regulates the gastric emptying rate through a feedback mechanism mediated by vagal nerves, and by physiological changes, such as gastric relaxation and the release of gastrointestinal hormones [3].

The overall process of digestion is coordinated by interactions between the gut and brain. Hunger is the sensation that leads us to seek and consume food, whereas satiety notifies us when to stop feeding.

Food intake is influenced by several types of gastrointestinal signals. These signals, when elicited by receptors in the stomach, provide information to the brain via the vagus nerve [6]. The stomach functions as a food reservoir; its capacity limits food intake. The gastric distention associated with ingestion of food activates tension mechanoreceptors and this generates a feeling of satiety. Pyloric chemoreceptors have an important role in regulating gastric motility, a fixed energy load being emptied into the duodenum at a constant rate regardless of meal composition. Conversely, gastrointestinal peptides, secreted by the stomach and small intestine with meals, primarily exert short–term effects on food intake. The gut peptides that reduce meal size are cholecystokinin (CCK), glucagon, glucagon – like peptide 1, amylin, somatostatin, peptide YY and bombesin. In contrast, ghrelin appears to have the opposite effect, stimulating enhanced food intake [3].

3. Pathophysiology of functional dyspepsia

Abnormal gastric motility and visceral hypersensitivity are thought to be the phenomena that are most closely related to the manifestation of FD symptoms.

Postprandial gastric motility may involve two possible sites: 1. the proximal stomach (fundus) exhibiting a disordered accommodation reflex after food ingestion, and/or 2. the antrum having abnormal gastric motor contractility. Proximal gastric distention, in fact, correlates very well with dyspeptic symptoms [2, 7]. The accommodation reflex is regarded as an appropriate response by which the stomach provides a reservoir facility for ingested food. In FD, this reflex can be impaired, leading to early satiety [8]. Such impairment occurs in 40 to 50% of FD patients [9]. In addition to impaired accommodation, delayed gastric emptying is also thought to contribute to the pathogenesis of FD. Food that is delayed in leaving the stomach provides the sensation that the stomach feels heavy. Some reports have suggested that delayed gastric emptying may be seen in up to 40% of FD patients [10].

Visceral hypersensitivity is also an important factor contributing to the feeling of dyspepsia. When a balloon is distended in the stomach of an FD patient, the threshold at which pain is perceived is significantly lower in FD patients compared to normal controls [11]. Such gastric hypersensitivity relates to symptoms of postprandial pain, belching and weight loss.

4. Nutrients and gastrointestinal function

Different nutrients and food items may modulate gastrointestinal motor and sensory functions, and so provoke gastrointestinal symptoms. The three basic nutritional components (carbohydrates, proteins and lipids) can contribute to disturbed gastrointestinal function. The individual nutritional components impact gastric emptying and the sensation of fullness differently. 1. Lipids (fat) and proteins exert a negative ("braking") effect on gastric motility. Fat releases enteric hormones (such as CCK) that increase pyloric sphincter tone and delay gastric emptying. 2.

Proteins alter gastric motility, leading to a feeling of fullness and this provides satiety. 3.

Carbohydrates and some food chemicals (like salicylates and amines) give rise to an osmotic effect with increased luminal volume. This can result in a sensation of fullness particularly in patients with visceral hypersensitivity.

In addition to the individual nutrients, the caloric content, the physical form, and the ingested volume of food affect the sensation of satiety and fullness. High meal viscosity has a greater effect on the sense of satiety, whereas high caloric foods delay gastric emptying. [12,13].

Dietary nutrients influence gastrointestinal function and seem to be related to symptom generation. Thus, it seems logical that disturbances of gastrointestinal motor and sensory functions can lead to generation of gastrointestinal symptoms after food ingestion. However, usually mixtures of food items are eaten, creating difficulties when attempting to pinpoint the individual responsible factor and limiting advice in terms of dietary restrictions in patients with dyspepsia. Dietary measures are classically prescribed in the management of patients with motility disorders, although they have not been systematically studied.

5. Role of meals in the generation of symptoms in functional dyspepsia

Epidemiologic studies, both in the USA and Europe, have shown that 50 to 80% of subjects with functional dyspepsia indicate that their symptoms are meal-related [5]. Meal ingestion is associated with diverse changes in the environment of the gastrointestinal lumen, the gastrointestinal function and potential physiopathological mechanisms. The two most cited causes of pathology are delayed gastric emptying and visceral hypersensitivity. After ingestion of a meal, patients with functional dyspepsia experience a marked rise in the intensity of their symptoms (epigastric burning, epigastric pain, fullness, bloating, nausea and belching) that persists for 4 hours [14]. Postprandial fullness is the most severe symptom that a meal aggravates.

Disturbances in upper gastrointestinal motor functions in FD have received considerable attention. Not surprisingly, current treatments such as prokinetics are primarily directed to these abnormalities. Therapies for visceral hypersensitivity remain difficult to establish. Factors such as eating patterns (meal size and frequency, nutrient composition, overall energy intake) and intolerances to specific foods or food groups have received little attention so far.

6. Dietary factors in functional dyspepsia

6.1. Eating patterns

Patients with functional dyspepsia frequently report that they are able to tolerate only small quantities of food [15], suggesting that their eating patterns differ from healthy subjects [8]. As a result of eating smaller quantities of food with lower energy intake, over half of FD patients experience weight loss even with a tendency to snack [16]. Despite eating fewer meals and consuming less total energy and fat, patients with FD experience fullness that is directly related to the amount of fat ingested and overall energy intake, while inversely related to the amount of carbohydrates ingested. Management of FD patients therefore might be improved by consuming smaller meals with reduced fat content [17,18].

6.2. Food intolerances

Patients with functional dyspepsia appear to exhibit more food intolerances than healthy persons, although studies are limited.

The belief that food is causing or at least triggering gut symptoms has led to the application of investigations purporting to guide dietary design. Various tests for food "intolerances" are widely available, such as skin prick (allergy) tests and assays for food specific immunoglobulins, but their value is unknown. Furthermore, various diets including wheat-free, anti-candida, carbohydrate-free, and other complex exclusions diets are touted in books and on the internet but evidence for any benefit is lacking.[19] The exception is the gluten-free diet, which will be discussed later in the chapter.

Alternative health practitioners and some nutritionists have advocated many such diets and intolerance-testing.

Therefore, gastroenterologists often are left with a defensive role when patients request dietary interventions. Although gastroenterologists may appreciate that food is an undoubted trigger, it is difficult to recognize the specific food item. Tests designed to this have a poor predictive value, while the resulting diets are often overly restrictive with the potential to render the patient nutritionally compromised [20].

How Food Triggers Gastrointestinal Symptoms?

The enteric nervous system is a major controller of multiple gut functions, such as secretion, motility, blood flow and mucosal growth. In a normal situation, low intensity stimuli from the lumen have few discernible effects on motility (as occurs in association with minimal inflation of the balloon during barostat studies).

In most patients with functional gastrointestinal disorders, there is a change in relationship between stimulus intensity and perception (the hallmark of visceral hypersensitivity) and efferent motility response. These people experience pain in response to low intensity stimuli; abnormal motility responses may ensue.

Luminal events may be initiated via two main stimuli: mechanical (associated with distention of the gut wall) and chemical stimuli. Chemical stimuli trigger specific enteroendocrine cells of the gut, releasing serotonin, which stimulates primary afferents of the enteric nervous system [21]. There is also evidence that some enteric neurons might directly respond to mechanical stimuli: the transient receptor potential (TRP) cation channels seem to be involved in most levels of control of gastrointestinal function, including visceral hypersensitivity [22]. The TRPV1 (vanilloid) channels appear to be central to the initiation and persistence of visceral hypersensitivity in an animal model. Increased expression of TRPV1 channels in neurons of the gut has been observed in patients with IBS; such expression correlates with visceral hypersensitivity, and with abdominal pain [23,24].

Food stimulates the gut through the release of enteric hormones and particularly via the enteric nervous system. A primary trigger is luminal distention, which results from the physical act of ingesting food and from secondary events such as gas production (especially bacterial fermentation). Food also contains potent chemicals. If the food constituents that stimulate the enteric nervous system were to be identified, then these would become obvious targets for dietary manipulation.

On the basis of these concepts (luminal distention, visceral hypersensitivity and chemical stimuli of the enteric nervous system), three specific areas of proven or suspected food-induced gut symptoms in patients with functional GI symptoms are important: a. FODMAPs (fermentable oligo-, di- and monosaccharides and polyols) that include luminal distention; b. food chemicals (salicylates, amines) that potentially stimulates the enteric nervous system (ENS), and c. gluten that may trigger symptoms by as yet unknown mechanisms.

a. *Targeting luminal distention: The FODMAP approach*

Carbohydrates occur across a range of foods regularly consumed including grains such as wheat and rye, vegetables, fruit and legumes. Short-chain carbohydrates with chain lengths up to 10 sugars vary in their digestibility and subsequent absorption. Those that are poorly absorbed exert osmotic effects in the intestinal lumen increasing its water volume. They are also rapidly fermented by bacteria yielding consequent gas production. These two effects may underlie many of the gastrointestinal symptoms that follows their ingestion. Only monosaccharides (glucose, galactose) can be actively absorbed across the small intestinal epithelium.

Di- and oligosaccharides must be hydrolyzed to their constituent hexoses for absorption to occur. All these molecules are plentiful in the diet and have been termed FODMAPs[1]

FODMAPs are therefore poorly absorbed, highly osmotic and rapidly fermented by gastrointestinal bacteria, leading to increased water and gas. The result is intestinal distention that also effects changes in motility, leading to symptoms of bloating and discomfort [26]. FOPMAPs induce functional symptoms in patients with IBS who have fructose malabsorption; reduction of dietary FODMAPs produces a durable symptomatic response [27, 28].

Some common food sources of FODMAPs are summarized in table 1:

	Oligosaccharides, fructans	Lactose	Fructose	Polyols
Fruit	Peach, persimmon, watermelon		Apple, cherry, mango, pear, Watermelon	Apple, apricot, pear, avocado, cherry, blackberries, plum, prune, nectarine
Vegetables	Artichokes, beetroot, Brussels sprouts, chicory, garlic, onion, peas		Asparagus, artichokes, sugar snap peas	Cauliflower, mushroom, snow peas
Grains , cereals	Wheat , rye, barley			
Nuts	pistachios			
Milk		Milk, yoghurt, ice-cream, custard, soft cheeses		
Legumes	Lentils, chickpeas			
Other	Chicory drinks		Honey, high fructose corn syrup	
Food additives	Inulin			Sorbitol, mannitol, maltitol, xylitol, isomalt

Table 1.

b. *Targeting food chemicals*

Plants produce a wide variety of chemicals, some of which have survival function (the bad taste for protection, odors for reproduction), along with antibacterial or preservative properties.

Potentially bioactive chemicals include salicylates (that have a protective role), amines and glutamates (that are products of protein breakdown), and common food additives such as benzoates, sulfites and, nitrates (as preservatives).

1 FODMAP is an acronym for different carbohydrates: F: fermentable; O: oligosaccharides (fructans , galacto-oligosaccharides); D: disaccharides (lactose); M: monosaccharides (fructose); A: and P: polyols (sorbitol , mannitol , xylitol , maltitol) [25].

In general, the stronger the flavor of the food, the higher the chemical content will be. In clinical practice, food chemicals have received some attention in the pathogenesis and management of urticaria, headaches, asthma and anaphylactic reactions.

Food chemicals are major afferent stimuli to the enteric nervous system. In the presence of visceral hypersensitivity, normal physiological stimulation by such chemicals might result in exaggerated effector responses (luminal distention). [32] Plant chemicals are able to activate TRP channels. Chronic exposure to certain chemicals will lead to increased expression of TRP channels and this contributes to a higher sensitivity of the enteric nervous system, and thus to the development of functional gut symptoms. Withdrawing the offending chemicals from the diet may reverse the TRP channel overexpression with subsequent resolution of the gut symptoms.

The only food chemicals that have been systematically studied with respect to gut symptoms are salicylates and related molecules such as non-steroid anti-inflammatory drugs. 2 to 4 % of patients with irritable bowel syndrome (IBS) or food allergies are salicylate-drug intolerant [29]. Examples of food sources containing high amounts of potentially bioactive chemicals are summarized in Table 2.

	Salicylates	Amines	Glutamates
Fruits	Avocado, berries , cherry, citrus , date, grape , kiwifruit, pineapple, plum , strawberry	Redcurrant	Dried prunes, raisins, grapes, plum, sultanas
Vegetables	Mushrooms, sauerkraut, spinach, tomato, chicory, eggplant, onion, chili, ginger, herbs	Eggplant, olives	
Grains , cereals	Breakfast cereals , mueslis, dried fruit, honey, coconut, potato chips		
Nuts	Almond, hazelnut, marzipan , peanut butter , nut pasta		
Seeds	Mustard seeds, sesame seed pasta		
Milk , milk products	Milk with chocolate, strawberry or banana flavor , yoghurt	Brie , camembert, parmesan , tasty cheeses	Brie , camembert , parmesan
Legumes	Bean mixes , broad beans , canned baked beans in sauce	Surimi, soy sauce , miso, tempeh	Canned baked beans in sauce , textured vegetable protein

	Salicylates	Amines	Glutamates
Meat, fish , chicken	Beef : smoked , corned , dried Chicken : nuggets , smoked Meat pastes , fish pastes , salami	Ham , bacon , anchovies, prawns tuna , fish : pickled , salted, smoked	Beef : billong, jerky Chicken : pressed , seasoned , gravy
Fats and oils	Almond oil , extra virgin olive oil , sesame , avocado oil	Almond oil , extra virgin olive oil , sesame oil	Almond oil , extra virgin olive oil , sesame oil
Beverages	Flavored mineral waters, spirits (except gin, tonic, whisky, vodka) , wine, fruit juices, ginger beer, beer , champagne , cider , herbal tea , tea	Beer , champagne , cider , tea , herbal tea , wine Chocolate drinks , cocoa powder	Beer , champagne , cider , tea , herbal tea , wine
Other	Jam , marmalade , fruit flavored syrup , yeast extract , vinegar (cider , red and white wine) Honey , peppermints, tomato sauce , soy sauce	Jam , marmalade , yeast extract , vinegar , chocolate , sauces ,	Jam , fruit flavored sweets , yeast extract , fermented products , chicken salt , sauces (tomato , soy , fish and oyster)

Table 2. Examples of food sources with very high amounts of salicylates, amines and glutamates (reference: http:// www.allergy.net.eu)

c. *Targeting gluten: A suspected molecule without a known mechanism*

A. *Celiac disease* in recent years has undergone a profound revision. Celiac disease (CD) is now considered to be a systemic immune-mediated disorder elicited by gluten. The common denominator for all patients with CD is the presence of a combination of gluten-dependent clinical manifestations, specific autoantibodies (anti–tissue transglutaminase, anti-endomysial antibodies plus serum IgA) and different degrees of enteropathy, ranging from lymphocytic infiltration of the epithelium to complete villous atrophy. [33, 34] Nevertheless, CD remains underdiagnosed in all age groups. The advent of serological testing has improved the detection of celiac disease but typical endoscopic findings for villous atrophy such as scalloping of folds, a mosaic pattern, or decreased folds are often not evident in less severe cases. Magnification tools like confocal endomicroscopy or "water immersion" techniques help characterize the abnormal duodenal mucosa and target biopsying. In many patients, particular adults, the disease features atypical symptoms or is completely silent, the so-called "celiac iceberg". Upper abdominal symptoms, such as abdominal pain and dyspepsia, are a common primary complaint in CD [36]. 30 to 40 % of celiac patients have dyspeptic symptoms. From a different perspective, diagnostic testing for celiac disease in individuals with dyspepsia has some advocates, because of a trend to a greater prevalence [35]. Nevertheless, the prevalence of biopsy-proven celiac disease in individuals with dyspepsia may be as low as 1%, a value similar to that amongst individuals in the general population, or markedly higher at 6% to 9% [37]. Routine screening for celiac disease therefore seems useful through serological testing and with distal duodenal biopsy during upper gastrointestinal endoscopy done to investigate dyspepsia.

B. *Gluten (wheat) sensitivity*. Gluten may also induce other pathological conditions, such as a wheat allergy. Wheat allergy is an immunoglobulin IgE–mediated disease and thus completely unrelated to celiac disease. [33] Recent attention however has been given to another entity: gluten or wheat sensitivity (also termed non-celiac gluten sensitivity). This disorder misses one or more of the key criteria: enteropathy and the presence of specific autoantibodies that define celiac disease (CD). The current working definition of non-celiac gluten sensitivity is the occurrence of irritable bowel syndrome (IBS)-like symptoms after ingesting gluten, and improvement after gluten withdrawal from the diet. Celiac disease must be excluded by negative celiac serology or a normal intestinal architecture, while wheat allergy should be negated by a negative IgE-mediated allergy test to wheat. Non-celiac gluten sensitivity (NCGS) thus encompasses a collection of medical conditions in which gluten leads to an adverse food reaction, clinically similar to some features of celiac disease, but celiac testing is negative or inconclusive [38, 39]. Such non-celiac IBS patients, in whom celiac disease is excluded, will improve on a gluten-free diet [30].

The key question is the mechanism by which gluten induces symptoms. Gluten may mediate cholinergic activation, leading to increased smooth muscle contractility and indirectly have effects on luminal water content. Another explanation might be the release of neutrally active peptides from the gluten digestion that might potentially gain access to enteric nerve endings. Gluten ingestion can precipitate duodenal tissue eosinophilia in those with wheat sensitivity [39]. Although there is no well-established mechanism for NCGS, the gluten-free diet has gained substantial popularity with the general public.

7. Dietary management strategies in functional dyspepsia

Because of the many patients with functional dyspepsia and its serious impairment to their quality of life, this entity represents an important clinical challenge. Pharmacologic therapies are limited, leaving patients and physicians to often use dietary strategies in managing FD.

Unfortunately most of the available information concerning the role of diet and food intake in FD patients is inconclusive. Several studies fortunately have shown clear differences between FD patients and healthy persons in the ability to tolerate certain types of foods including fermentable carbohydrates (FODMAPs).

FD patients often maintain regular consumption of several foods despite these being implicated with the dyspepsia. Why these patients do not avoid the majority of food components, which they link to dyspepsia, remains unclear. Possible reasons might be ignorance of this association, a lack of alternatives to replace food items, or cultural habits such as the use of coffee in some populations. Nevertheless dietary recommendations are intrinsic for managing FD. General advice should include consuming small, frequent meals that have a low-fat content.

Although such recommendations are helpful, specific strategies more commonly become necessary.

A well-trained nutritionist should direct the patient to record a 7-day food and symptom diary. It is also important to record other variables such as stress levels and activity as these factors can also impact symptomatology. The role of the dietitian is to explain the physiological basis of the diet, provide a list of suitable alternative foods and so restrict specific FODMAPs, while promoting a nutritionally adequate diet.

A low FODMAP diet is currently the first approach for many dietitians. This relatively complex diet involves the reduction, but not the complete avoidance of FODMAPs. Foods have been classified into high and low FODMAP content, and therefore knowledge of the FODMAP status of foods is an important skill for patient education (see table below). Low FODMAP foods that are suitable alternatives to foods high in FODMAP are encouraged. For example, rather than completely restricting fruit, reduce the intake of high FODMAP fruit and encourage the intake of FODMAP fruit [32]. After 6 to 8 weeks, the dietitian should undertake a review. If there is a satisfactory improvement, then a re-challenge could be done. It is important to determine the tolerance level, and also to increase variety in the diet. If the improvement is partial or absent, than additional dietary triggers should be emphasized: avoidance of some food chemicals such as salicylates, amines and glutamates, and last but not least a gluten-free diet might be initiated.

Any diet that aims to reduce one group of components will affect other dietary components with the potential to influence the same end point. This is certainly the case with a low FODMAP diet. As gluten-containing cereals also contain a high FODMAP content, any reduction of gluten intake would be accompanied by a decrease in other potentially symptom-inducing, cereal-related proteins. Likewise, if lactose is avoided in a proportion of patients, then the intake of dairy-associated proteins concomitantly may be reduced.

Type of food	**HIGH in FODMAP**	**LOW in FODMAP**
Milk	Milk : cow, sheep, goat, soy Creamy soups with milk Evaporated milk Sweetened condensed milk	Milk : almond, coconut, hazelnut, rice Lactose free cow's milk Lactose free ice cream
Yoghurt	Cow's milk yoghurt Soy yoghurt	Coconut milk yoghurt
Cheese	Cottage cheese Ricotta cheese Mascarpone cheese	Hard cheeses : cheddar, Swiss, brie, blue cheese, mozzarella, parmesan, feta No more than 2 tablespoons ricotta or cottage cheese

Type of food	HIGH in FODMAP	LOW in FODMAP
		Lactose free cottage cheese
Dairy-based condiments	Sour cream Whipping cream	Butter Cream cheese
Dairy-based desserts	Ice cream Frozen yoghurt Sherbet	Sorbet from FODMAPs friendly fruit
Fruit	Apples, pears Cherries , raspberries, blackberries Watermelon Nectarines, white peaches, apricots, plums Peaches Prunes Mango, papaya Persimmon Orange fruit Canned fruit Large portions of any fruit	Banana Blueberries, strawberries Cantaloupe, honeydew Grapefruit, lemon, lime Grapes Kiwi Pineapple Rhubarb Tangelos <1/4 avocado <1 tablespoon dried fruit Consume ripe fruit ; less-ripe fruit contains more fructose
Vegetables	Artichokes Asparagus Sugar snap peas Cabbage Onions Shallot Leek Onion and garlic salt powders Garlic Cauliflower Mushrooms Pumpkin Green peppers	Bok choy , bean sprouts Red bell pepper Lettuce, spinach Carrots Chives, spring onion Cucumber Eggplant Green beans Tomato Potatoes Garlic infused oil Water chestnuts <1 stick celery <1/2 cup sweet potato, broccoli, Brussels sprouts
Grains	Wheat Rye Barley-large quantities Spelt	Brown rice Oats , oat bran Quinoa Corn Gluten-free bread, cereals , pastas and crackers without honey Apple/pear juice , agave

Type of food	HIGH in FODMAP	LOW in FODMAP
Legumes	Chickpeas , hummus Kidney beans, baked beans Soy milk Lentils	Tofu Peanuts <1/3 cup green peas
Nuts and seeds	Pistachios	1-2 tablespoons almonds, pecans, pine nuts, walnuts, sunflower seeds, sesame seeds
Sweeteners	Honey Agave High fructose corn syrup Sorbitol, mannitol, xylitol, maltitol	Sugars Glucose , sucrose Pure maple syrup Aspartame
Additives	Inulin Fructose-oligosaccharides Sugar alcohols Chicory root	
Alcohol	Rum	Wine , beer Vodka , gin
Protein-rich food		Fish, chicken, turkey, eggs, meat

Table 3. FODMAP status of food

8. Summary

Functional dyspepsia is a clinical problem of considerable magnitude for the health care system due to its high prevalence and the chronic or recurrent nature of symptoms. The manifestation of FD symptoms is directly caused by physiological abnormalities: abnormal gastroduodenal motility and/or visceral hypersensitivity. The therapeutic options for a clinician are limited and far from optimal: pharmacological therapies often fail. As food ingestion commonly triggers gastrointestinal symptoms, a dietary approach would seem most effective. There is reasonable evidence to suggest that a low FODMAP diet is beneficial, while gluten sensitivity may benefit others particularly in patients with IBS features. Gastroenterologists should no longer ignore specific dietary intervention for patients with functional dyspepsia.

Author details

Jan Pen

H. Hartziekenhuis – Lier, Department of Internal Medicine, Division of gastroenterology, Belgium

References

[1] Tack J., Bisschops R.: Mechanisms underlying meal-induced symptoms in functional dyspepsia. Gastroenterology, 2204, Dec 127 (6): 1844-1847

[2] Miwa H. Why dyspepsia can occur without organic disease: pathogenesis and management of functional dyspepsia. J. Gastroenterology, 2012, Aug, 47 (8): 862-871

[3] Karamanolis G., Tack J. Nutrition and motility disorders. Best Practice and Research Clin. Gastroenterol., 2006 ; 20 (3): 485-505

[4] Feinle-Bisset C., Horowitz M. Dietary factors in functional dyspepsia. Neurogastroenterology. Motility, 2006, 18: 608-618

[5] Feinle-Bisset C., Vozzo R., Horowitz M., Talley N. Diet, food intake and disturbed physiology in the pathogenesis of symptoms in functional dyspepsia. Am J Gastroenterol 2004, Jan 99 (1): 170-181

[6] Wood S.C. Gastrointestinal satiety signals. An overview of gastrointestinal signals that influences food intake. Am J Physiol Gastrointest Liver Physiol. 2004, 286: G7-G13

[7] Thumshirm M. Pathophysiology of functional dyspepsia. Gut 2002, 51 (Suppl 1): 3-66

[8] Tack J.,Piessevaux H., Coulie B., Caenepeel P.,Janssens J. Role of impaired gastric accommodation to a meal in functional dyspepsia. Gastroenterology 1998, 115: 1346-1352

[9] Tack J. Functional dyspepsia: impaired fundic accommodation. Curr Treat Options Gastroenterol, 2000, 3: 287-294

[10] Quartero A.O., de Wit N.J., Lodder A.C., Numans M.E., Smout A.J., Hoes A.W. Disturbed solid-phase gastric emptuying in non functional dyspepsia: a meta analysis. Dig Dis Sci 1998, 43: 2028-2033

[11] Lemann M., Dederding J.P., Flourie B., Franchisseur C., Rambaud J.C., Jian R. Abnormal perception of visceral pain in response to gastric distention in chronic idiopathic dyspepsia. The irritable stomach syndrome. Dig Dis Sci 1991, 36: 1241-1254

[12] Marciani L., Gowland P.A., Spiller P.C., Manoy P., Moore R.J., Young P., Fillery-Travis A.J. Effect of meal viscosity and nutrients on satiety, intragastric dilation and emptying assessed by MRI. Am J Gastrointest Liver Physiol 2001, 280: G1227-G1233

[13] Hill A.J., Blundell J.E. Macro-nutrients and satiety:the effects of a high protein or a high carbohydrate meal on subjective motivation to eat and food preferences. Nutr Behav 1986, 3: 133-144

[14] Bisschops R., Karamanolis G., Arts J., Caenepeel P, Verbeke K.,Janssens J., Tack J. Relationship between symptoms and ingestion of a meal in functional dyspepsia. Gut 2008, 57: 1495-1503

[15] Carvalho R.V., Lorena S.L.,Almeida J.R., Mesquita M.A. Food intolerance, diet composition and eating patterns in functional dyspepsia patients. Dig Dis Sci 2010, 55: 60-65

[16] Mullan A., Kavanagh P., O'Mahony P., Joy T., Gleeson F., Gibney M.J. Food and nutrients intakes and eating patterns in functional and organic dyspepsia. Eur J Clin Nutr 1994, 48: 97-105

[17] Pilichiewicz A.N., Horowitz M., Holtmann G.J., Talley N.J., Feinle-Bisset C. Relationship between symptoms and dietary patterns in patients with functional dyspepsia. Clin Gastroenterol Hepatol 2009, 7 (3): 317-322

[18] Talley N.J., Locke G.R., Lahr B.D., et al. Functional dyspepsia, delayed gastric emptying and impaired quality of life. Gut 2006, 55: 933-939

[19] Mullin G.E., Swift K.M., Lipski L. et al. Testing for food reactions: the good, the bad and the ugly. Nutr Clin Pract 2010, 25: 192-198

[20] Monsbakken K.W., Vandvik P.O, Farup P.G. Perceived food intolerance in subjects with irritable bowel syndrome: etiology, prevalence and consequences. Eur. J. Clin. Nutr. 2006 ; 60: 667-672.

[21] Sternini C., Anselmi L., Rozengurt E. Enteroendocrine cells: a site of "taste" in gastrointestinal chemosensing. Curr. Opin. Endocrinol. Diabetes Obes. 2008 ; 15: 73-78.

[22] Boesmans W., Busianik G., Tack J., et al. TRP channels in neurogastroenterology: opportunities for therapeutic interventions. Br. J. Pharmacol. 2011 ; 162: 18-37.

[23] Chan C.I., Faces P., Davis J.B. et al. Sensory fibres expressing capsaicin receptor TRPV1 in patients with rectal hypersensitivity and faecal urgency. Lancet 2003 ; 361: 385-391.

[24] Faces P. et al. Increased capsaicin receptor TRPV1 expressing sensory fibres in irritable bowel syndrome and their correlations with abdominal pain. Gut 2008 ; 57: 923-929.

[25] Gibson P.R., Shepherd S.J.. Personal view: food for thought-Western lifestyle and susceptibility for Crohn's disease. The FOPMAD hypothesis. Aliment. Pharmacol. Ther. 2005 ; 21: 1399-1409.

[26] Gibson P.R., Newnham E., Barrett J.S. et al. Review article: fructose malabsorption and the bigger picture. Aliment. Pharmacol. Ther. 2007 ; 25: 349-363.

[27] Shepherd S.J., Parker F.C., Muir J.G. et al. Dietary triggers of abdominal symptoms in patients with IBS: randomized placebo-controlled evidence. Clin. Gastroenterol. Hepatol. 2008 ; 6: 765-771.

[28] Gibson P.R., Shepherd S.J. Evidence-based dietary management of functional gastrointestinal symptoms: the FODMAP approach. J. Gastroenterol Hepatol ; 2010 ; 25: 252-258.

[29] Raithel M.,Baenkler H.W., Nayel A. et al. Significance of salicylate intolerance in diseases of the lower gastrointestinal tract. J. Physiol. Pharmacol. 2005 ; 56 (Suppl 5): 89-102.

[30] Biesiekierski J.R., Appl B., Newnham E.D., Irving P.M. et al. Gluten causes gastrointestinal symptoms in subjects without celiac disease: a double-blind randomized placebo-controlled trial. Am. J. Gastroenterol. 2011 ; 106: 508-514.

[31] Boettcher E., Crowe S.E. Dietary proteins and functional gastrointestinal disorders. Am. J. Gastroenterol. 2013 online publication 9 April 2013 ; doi 10.1038.

[32] Gibson P.R., Shepherd S.J. Food choice as a key management strategy for functional gastrointestinal symptoms. Am. J. Gastroenterol. 2012 ; 107: 657-666.

[33] Troncone R., Jabri B. Coeliac disease and gluten sensitivity. Journal of internal Medicine. 2011 ; 269: 582-590.

[34] Keshavarz A.A., Bashiri H., Ahmadi A, et al. The prevalence of occult celiac disease among patients with functional dyspepsia: a study from the western region of Iran. Gastrointestinal research and Practice. 2010 Article ID, 170702,4 pages.

[35] Giangreco E., D'agate C., Barbera C., et al. Prevalence of celiac disease in adult patients with refractory functional dyspepsia: value of routine duodenal biopsy. World J. Gastroenterol. 2008 ; 14 [45]: 6948-6953.

[36] Ehsani-Ardakani M.J., Nejad M.R., et al. Gastrointestinal and non-gastrointestinal presentation in patients with celiac disease. Archives of Iranian Medicine. 2013 ;16 (2): 78-82.

[37] Ford AC, Ching E, Moayyedi P. Meta-analysis: yield of diagnostic tests for coeliac disease in dyspepsia Aliment Pharmacol & Ther 2009;30(1): 28–36.

[38] Boettcher E, Crowe SE. Dietary proteins and functional gastrointestinal disorders. Am J Gastroenterol 2013; 108:728–736.

[39] Carroccio A, Mansueto P, Iacono G, et al. Non-celiac wheat sensitivity diagnosed by double-blind placebo-controlled challenge: Exploring a new clinical entity. Am J Gastroenterol 2012; 107:1898–1906

Chapter 7

Biliary Dyspepsia: Functional Gallbladder and Sphincter of Oddi Disorders

Meena Mathivanan, Liisa Meddings and
Eldon A. Shaffer

Additional information is available at the end of the chapter

http://dx.doi.org/10.5772/56779

1. Introduction

Biliary-type abdominal pain is common and often presents a clinical challenge for physicians. True biliary colic consists of episodes of steady pain across the right upper quadrant and epigastric regions, lasting from 30 minutes to 6 hours [1]. Such abdominal pain, when it lasts longer than 6 hours, is likely due to complications of gallstone disease such as acute cholecystitis or acute pancreatitis, or represents a non-biliary source of pain [1].

1.1. Cholelithiasis, biliary pain and atypical dyspepsia

Classical biliary pain that occurs in the setting of gallstones represents symptomatic cholelithiasis. The symptoms associated with gallstones however are frequently confusing. In fact, only 13% of people with gallstones ever develop biliary pain when followed for 15–20 years [2], meaning that most (70-90%) patients with gallstones never experience biliary symptoms. Vague dyspeptic complaints like belching, bloating, flatulence, heartburn and nausea are not characteristic for biliary disease [3, 4]. Therefore, it is not surprising that cholecystectomy often fails to relieve such ambiguous symptoms in those with documented gallstones. In fact, cholecystectomy fails to relieve symptoms in 10-33% of patients with documented gallstones [5]. If the abdominal pain is misdiagnosed and instead due to functional gut disorders like irritable bowel syndrome, cholecystectomy would not provide a favorable outcome [4, 5, 6].

1.2. Functional gallbladder disease

Biliary-type abdominal pain (also termed biliary colic) in the context of a structurally normal gallbladder has been referred to as "biliary dyspepsia". True biliary pain manifests as steady, severe epigastric or right upper quadrant pain that might radiate through to the back and right infrascapular regions, lasting for at least thirty minutes but less than 6 hours. It can be associated with symptoms of nausea and vomiting, and may awaken the patient from sleep [8]. Episodes are recurrent but usually in a sporadic and quite erratic frequency. Its functional nature should be supported by an absence of markers of organic disease: normal liver and pancreatic biochemistries, and negative diagnostic imaging. No structural basis should be evident to explain the pain.

Functional biliary pain has also been termed: *gallbladder dyskinesia, chronic acalculous gallbladder dysfunction, acalculous biliary disease* and *chronic acalculous cholecystitis [9].* "Biliary dyskinesia" implies a motility disorder resulting from abnormal motor function of the gallbladder (manifest as impaired emptying) and/or sphincter of Oddi (increased tone)[10].

1.3. Functional disorders of the biliary tract (Sphincter of Oddi dysfunction)

Following removal of the gallbladder, biliary pain has been attributed to sphincter of Oddi dysfunction (SOD). SOD represents intermittent obstruction to the flow of biliopancreatic secretions through the sphincter of Oddi in the absence of biliary stones or a ductal stricture [11]. The Rome III Consensus has developed criteria for functional biliary-type pain (Table 1) [8].

2. Epidemiology

Dyspepsia overall is a common symptom in the general population with reported prevalence rates ranging between 10-45% [12]. Such estimates are confounded by the use of differing criteria for defining dyspepsia as well as a recurrent failure to exclude patients who primarily report heartburn symptoms[12]. Nevertheless, dyspepsia remains a common issue with annual incidence rates estimated between 1-6%[13]. In the United States, there were 4,007,198 outpatient visits for gastroenteritis or dyspepsia and 130,744 hospital admissions for functional or motility disorders in 2009 [14]. This represents a 26% increase from the year 2000, which suggests an upsurge in the overall incidence of dyspepsia[14].

Epidemiology of functional gallbladder disease (i.e.; Frequency of biliary pain with a normal appearing gallbladder e.g. without gallstones)

The true prevalence of biliary dyspepsia is unknown. Estimates are generally based on the presence of non-specific clinical features and a lack of structural findings on ultrasonographic investigation of the biliary system. In large Italian population-based studies, 7.6% of men and 20.7% of women experienced biliary pain yet lacked gallstones on abdominal ultrasonography [15, 16].

With the advent of minimally invasive surgery, biliary dyskinesia has become a new indication for laparoscopic cholecystectomy increasing 348% in adults [17] and escalating 700% in pediatric patients over approximately a decade [18]. Large scale case series now list biliary

http://dx.doi.org/10.5772/56779

dyskinesia as the primary indication for cholecystectomy in 10-20% of adults [17, 19-22] and 10-50% of pediatric patients [23-26].

Epidemiology of functional sphincter of Oddi disorders (i.e.; Frequency of biliary pain after the gallbladder has been removed – postcholecystectomy).

In the US householder survey of presumably healthy adults, 69% expressed symptoms indicating a functional gastrointestinal syndrome within the previous three months and 1.5% had biliary dyspepsia following cholecystectomy [27]. Women were more commonly afflicted at 2.3% than men at 0.6% [27]. Nevertheless, sphincter of Oddi dysfunction (SOD) is uncommon in this population. SOD, when documented by ERCP manometry, occurs in less than 1% of the patients who have had their gallbladders removed and accounts for the abdominal pain in 14% of the patients with postcholecystectomy pain [28].

3. Pathophysiology

3.1. Acute biliary pain

The biliary tract normally is a low-pressure conduit though which bile secreted from the liver reaches the duodenum. The gallbladder acts as a reservoir for decompression while storing bile in the interdigestive periods overnight and throughout the day [29]. Even in the digestive phase, gallbladder contraction does not elicit marked pressure spikes within the biliary tree because the sphincter of Oddi effectively relaxes. The hormone cholecystokinin (CCK) is primarily responsible for this reciprocity.

In the setting of cholelithiasis, biliary pain is assumed to originate from either an obstructive event (the gallbladder contracting on a closed cystic duct which is blocked by a gallstone) that increases intrabiliary pressure and/or inflammation (cholecystitis)[10]. Such obstruction also appears to stimulate the gallbladder mucosa to produce a phospholipase, which then hydrolyses fatty acids off lecithin to yield lysolecithin in bile. Lysolecithin, acting as a biological detergent, might then initiate an inflammatory reaction (cholecystitis). Subsequently, inflammatory mediators could trigger painful stimuli, while mechanoreceptor afferent fibers in the gallbladder and biliary tree conduct visceral pain information to the spinal cord and the brain. Thus, motor contraction, sensory afferents producing painful sensations and obstruction/inflammation may all play a role in the perception of acute biliary-type pain.

3.2. Chronic functional biliary pain

The basis for chronic functional biliary pain appears to reside in visceral hypersensitivity, altered central processing, and/or abnormal gastrointestinal motility. Prolonged or intense noxious stimuli, particularly when repeated, lead to sensitization of visceral nociceptors. These peripheral sensory neurons respond to potentially damaging stimuli by sending nerve signals to the spinal cord (dorsal horn) and then projecting centrally to the brain – the thalamus and cortex, the site of pain perception. Chronic irritation might then influence afferent input and the release of neuroactive chemicals in the dorsal horn of the spinal cord. Even when the peripheral irritation ceases, synaptic changes in the spinal cord can persist, causing "pain memory". Thus, irritation to the biliary tract can potentially sensitize the nervous system. In some, the central nervous system becomes so sensitive that *hyperalgesia* results: severe pain evoked by only mildly painful stimuli. Persistent central excitability might subsequently result in *allodynia*: innocuous stimuli produce pain [30, 31]. Thus, the basis for abnormally heightened biliary sensations can reside at any level: either altered receptor sensitivity of the viscus, increased excitability of the neurons in the spinal cord dorsal horn, and/or altered central modulation of sensation, including psychological influences that affect the interpretation of these sensations. Further, central hyperexcitability can effect changes in the dorsal horn.

Acalculous biliary pain may represent a generalised motor disorder of the duct: the irritable gallbladder/sphincter of Oddi[10]. The abnormalities identified by impaired gallbladder emptying or increased tone in the sphincter of Oddi, for example, may reflect a more generalised motility disorder of the gut [32]. Moreover, biliary-type pain could originate from a neighbouring structure: for example, abnormal small intestinal motility. Gut smooth muscle in functional gut disorders exhibits altered sensitivity to regulatory peptides such as CCK, precipitating abdominal pain in some patients and confounding the interpretation of intestinal versus biliary pain.

Functional biliary disorders have been most prominently linked to abnormal motility of the gallbladder and/or sphincter of Oddi, in part because techniques exist to detect them in clinical practice. Biliary pain is construed to result in most instances from increased gallbladder pressure from either abnormal gallbladder contraction ("dyskinesia") and/or structural or functional outlet obstruction either at the exit from the gallbladder (e.g.; abnormal cystic duct) or at the sphincter of Oddi ("the fighting gallbladder"). Reduced emptying and pain however may also reflect diminished gallbladder contractility ("hypokinesia"). Decreased gallbladder emptying has been attributed to abnormal CCK release, decreased gallbladder CCK receptor sensitivity or density, or increased cystic duct receptor sensitivity to CCK with impaired smooth-muscle contractility producing outlet obstruction [33].

Impaired gallbladder emptying, however, is also an important pathogenetic component in cholesterol gallstones. Cholesterol gallstone formation begins when the liver produces bile supersaturated with cholesterol, in excess of the solubilizing agents, bile salts and lecithin. In this first stage, the liver secretes excess cholesterol into bile canaliculi that is accompanied by lecithin as small, unilamellar vesicles. These fuse in this supersaturated bile to become cholesterol-rich, multilamellar vesicles (liquid crystals). Aided by nucleating factors (biliary proteins), cholesterol microcrystals precipitate out of solution. Mucin, a glycoprotein, secreted by the gallbladder mucosa, then acts as a matrix scaffold to retain these cholesterol microcrystals. Diminished gallbladder contractility facilitates retention, providing the residence time that is necessary for these microcrystals to agglomerate and grow into overt gallstones. Cholesterol constitutes the vast majority (>85%) of gallstones. A minority of gallstones are black pigment stones. These are composed of calcium bilirubinate polymers that result from abnormal bilirubin metabolism. Such black pigment stones tend to develop in advanced age, Crohn's disease, extensive ileal resection, cirrhosis, cystic fibrosis, and chronic hemolytic states [34].

Hence, a smooth muscle defect producing gallbladder hypomotility is intrinsic to cholesterol gallstone formation and disease [35, 36] and also occurs in chronic acalculous disease [37]. Both conditions yield biliary pain, creating a potentially confusing scenario. Evidence of microlithiasis in the gallbladder bile in some patients with biliary dyskinesia [38] may merely indicate that excessive cholesterol, likely a stage of stone formation in which macroscopic gallstones were not evident, compromised signal transduction in the gallbladder and was the mechanism for reduced emptying. Certainly any bile crystals or sludge may eventually result in calculous disease, causing obstruction of the gallbladder and symptoms of biliary pain, but this must be distinguished from functional gallbladder disease. The mechanism for chronic cholecystitis is unclear [39], while cholesterolosis with its accumulation of lipid products (triglycerides and cholesterol precursors and esters) is likely too common to have any clinical importance as a cause of biliary pain [38].

Gallbladder dysmotility is also associated with other conditions including functional gastrointestinal disorders, pregnancy, diabetes mellitus, obesity, cirrhosis [40], and the use of various medications (including atropine, morphine, octreotide, nifedipine, and progesterone) [41]. Interestingly, gut smooth muscle in the irritable bowel syndrome (IBS) also exhibits altered sensitivity to regulatory peptides such as CCK [42]. It is, therefore, not surprising that the gallbladder empties abnormally in some patients with IBS [43-45].

Although in sphincter of Oddi dysfunction, pain has classically been attributed to abnormal smooth muscle motility, there may also be a component of visceral hypersensitivity. Here, the hypersensitivity might arise in a structure adjacent to the sphincter, the duodenum [46, 47].

3.3. Biliary dyspepsia and fatty food intolerance

Despite biliary dyspepsia suggesting impaired digestion, there is no consistent relationship to eating. Historically, the abdominal discomfort and bloating that follow a heavy, fatty meal has been termed "fatty food" intolerance, connoting an association between fat content in the diet and biliary dyspepsia [48, 49, 59]. Patients with biliary dyspepsia may eat fewer meals, perhaps because their symptoms onset after eating [51]. In some, the sensation of fullness experienced relates to the amount of fat consumed. The presumed basis is fat releasing CCK and peptide YY, which are gut hormones important in regulating hunger and satiety. Patients with biliary dyspepsia, particularly those experiencing higher scores for nausea and pain, have higher concentrations of fasting and postprandial CCK compared to healthy individuals[50]. However, just as dyspepsia is not a particular manifestation of gallstone disease, fatty foods do not necessarily precipitate attacks of biliary colic [3, 52].

4. Differential diagnoses

Structural causes affecting the gastrointestinal tract should be considered in any patient presenting with dyspepsia (Table 2) [12]. Gallstones, biliary sludge and microlithiasis must be eliminated [12]. As decreased gallbladder emptying is a key investigation leading to the diagnosis of a functional gallbladder disorder, other causes of impaired gallbladder emptying should be identified to obviate confounders (Table 3) [53].

Must include episodes of pain located in the epigastrium and/or right upper quadrant and all of the following:
1. Episodes lasting 30 minutes or longer
2. Recurrent symptoms occurring at different intervals (not daily)
3. The pain builds up to a steady level
4. The pain is moderate to severe enough to interrupt the patient's daily activities or lead to an emergency department visit
5. The pain is not relieved by bowel movements
6. The pain is not relieved by postural change
7. The pain is not relieved by antacids
8. Exclusion of other structural disease that would explain the symptoms
Supportive criteria:
The pain may present with 1 or more of the following:
1. Pain is associated with nausea and vomiting
2. Pain radiates to the back and/or right infrasubscapular region
3. Pain awakens from sleep in the middle of the night

Table 1. Rome III Diagnostic Criteria for Functional Gallbladder and Sphincter of Oddi Disorders [8]

Gastrointestinal Disorders
Gastroesophageal reflux disease
Gastric or esophageal cancer
Gastric infections
Gastroparesis
Inflammatory bowel disease
Irritable bowel syndrome
Peptic ulcer disease
Food intolerances
Drug intolerances
Pancreaticobiliary Disorders
Cholelithiasis, choledocholithiasis
Pancreatitis
Pancreatic neoplasms
Systemic Disorders
Adrenal insufficiency
Diabetes mellitus
Hyperparathyroidism
Renal insufficiency
Thyroid disease

Table 2. Organic Causes for Dyspepsia [12]

Primary gallbladder disease	
	Cholesterol gallstones
	Prior to stone formation as evidenced by microcrystals of cholesterol and following medical dissolution
	Pigment stones
	Hemoglobinopathies
	Cholecystitis
	Acute or chronic, with or without stones
Metabolic disorders	
	Obesity, diabetes, pregnancy, VIPoma, sickle hemoglobinopathy
Neuromuscular defects	
	Myotonia dystrophic Denervation (spinal cord injury, vagotomy)
Functional gastrointestinal diseases: functional dyspepsia, functional abdominal pain	
	Irritable bowel syndrome
Deficiency of cholecystokinin	
	Celiac disease, fasting/TPN
Drugs	
	Anticholinergic agents, calcium channel blockers, opioids, ursodeoxycholic acid, octreotide, cholecystokinin-A receptor antagonist, nitric oxide donors, female sex hormones (progestins)

Table 3. Causes of Impaired Gallbladder Emptying [52]

5. Diagnosis

The diagnosis of functional disorders of the gallbladder and sphincter of Oddi should be based on the Rome III criteria for functional gallbladder and sphincter of Oddi disorders (Table 1).

5.1. Functional gallbladder disease

1. Preliminary investigations to rule out structural disease that might be the origin of the pain must include liver and pancreatic biochemistries and esophagogastroduodenoscopy. All should be normal in functional gallbladder disorder. The search for gallstones must be scrupulous. Transabdominal ultrasound is critical in being capable of detecting stones down to 3-5 mm in size. Endoscopic ultrasound (EUS) is more refined for microlithiasis: tiny stones < 3mm and biliary sludge [10]. Microscopic examination of gallbladder bile collected from the duodenum following IV CCK stimulation can detect deposits, either cholesterol as birefringent crystals (Figure 1) or pigment in the form of dark red-brown

calcium bilirubinate. Both techniques are fairly specific (in the order of 90%). Detection of microlithiasis by EUS however is more sensitive (96% versus 67%) than microscopic bile examination [54, 55], and also more available in most centres. Regardless, the use of these investigations in biliary dyskinesia is limited by their invasive nature.

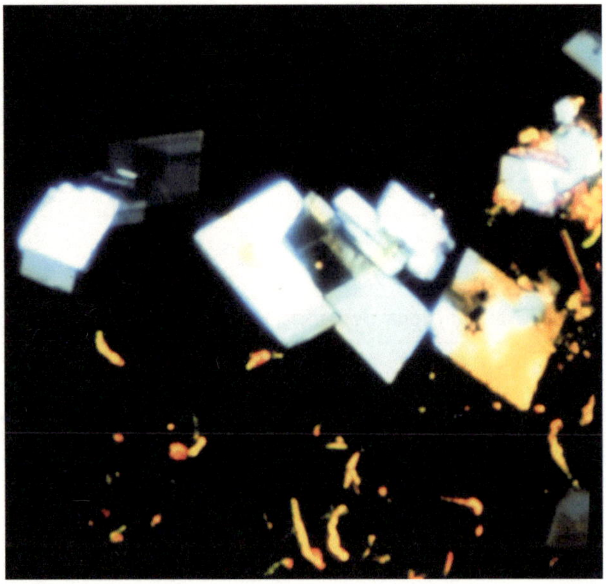

Figure 1. Cholesterol microcrystals in aspirated duodenal bile following CCK stimulation. The collected golden brown duodenal bile is first centrifuged and then examined under polarizing microscopy. As seen here, cholesterol is evident as birefringent, rhomboid-shaped crystals, characteristically with a notch in one corner.

2. Assessment of gallbladder emptying by cholecystokinin-cholescintigraphy is currently the key to diagnosing functional gallbladder disorder. The gallbladder ejection fraction (GBEF) is best measured via a nuclear medicine hepatobiliary scan. The radiopharmaceutical, technetium 99m-labelled iminodiacetic acid (HIDA), when infused intravenously, is readily taken up by hepatocytes, excreted into the bile, and accumulates in the gallbladder [37, 56, 57]. Infusion of the CCK analogue, Sincalide™ (the 8-amino acid C-terminal fragment of cholecystokinin, CCK-8), then initiates gallbladder evacuation (Figure 2). There has been a wide variation in methodology, leading to a consensus recommendation: Sincalide™ should be infused at 0.02μg/kg over 60 minutes. Normal gallbladder ejection fraction should be ≥ 38%, according to a recent consensus conference [58]. In selected cases of recurrent biliary pain in which no structural cause is evident, no stone disease is apparent and there exists no other associated cause for impaired gallbladder emptying, cholecystectomy is a reasonable consideration when the gallbladder ejection fraction is reduced at less than 35-40% [59].

http://dx.doi.org/10.5772/56779

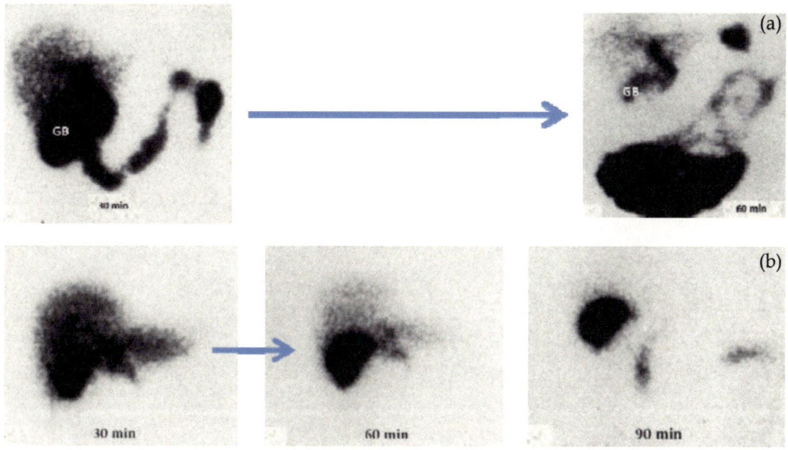

Figure 2. A. Normal gallbladder emptying on CCK-cholescintigraphy. The gallbladder is visualized 30 minutes after the injection of the 99m-labelled technetium iminodiacetic acid radiopharmaceutical (HIDA scan). Cholecystokinin is then infused (shown as arrow). Prompt gallbladder emptying (70% here) then ensues with the radiolabel ejected into the small intestine. The gallbladder is depicted as GB, before and after the CCK infusion. [52], B. Abnormal gallbladder emptying. Although the gallbladder fills, becoming well visualized at 30 minutes, the CCK infusion (arrow) has little effect thirty minutes later at 60 minutes into the study or even with an additional thirty minutes at 90 minutes. The liver washes out during this period of time. [52]

There is as yet no predictive value for CCK-cholescintigraphy in those with established yet uncomplicated ('silent") gallstones. The influence of gallbladder evacuation on the development of biliary symptoms and on the severity of disease remains unclear [56]. The sluggish gallbladder does not protect an individual with stones from developing pain.

The use of a fatty meal to stimulate gallbladder contraction may be more physiological and cheaper than CCK but does not enjoy an established protocol with normal values. Another limitation is that endogenous CCK release depends upon gastric emptying of the meal; gastroparesis often accompanies functional gastrointestinal disorders [58].

Real-time ultrasound has also been used to measure volume changes as the gallbladder empties. Its advantage over a nuclear medicine scan obviates exposing the patient to ionizing radiation. Quantitative ultrasonography, based on geometric assumptions, however is operator-dependent, limiting its accuracy. Although 3-dimensional and 4-dimensional ultrasounds appear to correlate reasonably well with HIDA scans in identifying reduced gallbladder ejection fractions [60], CCK-cholescintigraphy is more precise and remains the standard [56, 58, 60].

The CCK-provocation test aimed to reproduce the biliary pain following an infusion of CCK, implicating the gallbladder as the culprit. This test has fallen out of favor due to lack of objectivity and specificity for biliary dyskinesia [42, 61]. Rapid infusion of CCK can elicit abdominal pain even in normal individuals [10].

The algorithm for diagnosing and managing functional gallbladder disorder is outlined in Figure 3 [8].

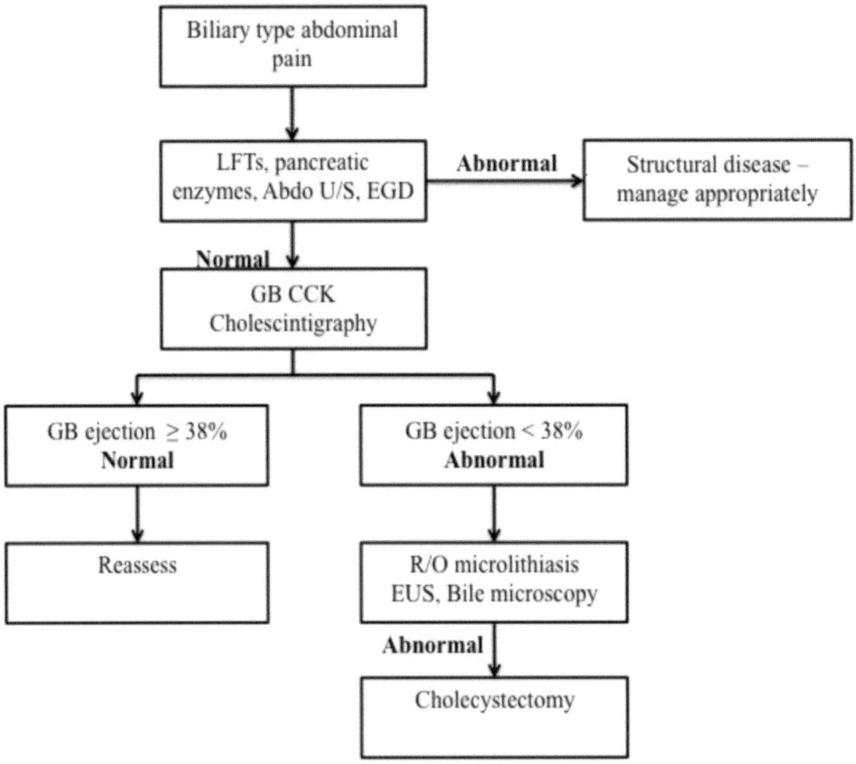

Figure 3. Algorithm for the diagnostic workup and management for biliary dyspepsia due to functional gallbladder disorder [8]. Patients with biliary type abdominal pain should initially undergo non-invasive investigations including relevant laboratory work and an abdominal ultrasound. An endogastroduodenoscopy (EGD) should then be performed and if any structural abnormalities, should be treated by medical, endoscopic or surgical management. A gallbladder cholecystokinin (GB CCK) cholescintigraphy can be subsequently performed. If there is abnormal ejection, EUS (endoscopic ultrasound) or bile microscopy can be used to further investigate for microlithiasis. Even in the absence of microlithiasis, if the ejection fraction is abnormal on GB CCK cholescintigraphy and no obvious confounding factor identified, consider referring the patient for a cholecystectomy.

5.2. Functional Sphincter of Oddi Disorder (SOD)

Sphincter of Oddi dysfunction implies that the basis is a motility disorder of the sphincter that intermittently results in pain, elevated liver and/or pancreatic enzymes, a dilated common duct and potentially pancreatitis. The Milwaukee classification originally categorizes SOD into three types, separating functional biliary and pancreatic sphincter of Oddi disorders on the basis of symptoms, laboratory tests and radiological imaging [8, 62-65] (Table 4). As these require an invasive procedure, endoscopic cholangiopancreatography (ERCP), to measure common duct size and biliary drainage, the criteria have been revised to use non-invasive imaging for estimating duct size of on an abdominal ultrasound [64].

http://dx.doi.org/10.5772/56779

Biliary type
Type I:
Typical biliary type pain Liver enzymes (AST, ALT or ALP) > 2 times normal limit documented on at least 2 occasions during episodes of pain Dilated CBD > 8 mm in diameter Positive manometry for biliary SOD (seen in 65-95% of patients)
Type II:
Biliary type pain and one of the above criteria (laboratory or imaging)
Type III:
Biliary type pain only
Pancreatic type SOD
Type I:
Pancreatic type pain Amylase and/or lipase > 2 times upper normal limit on at least 2 occasions during episodes of pain Dilated pancreatic duct (head > 6 mm, body > 5 mm)
Type II:
Pancreatic type pain, and one of the above criteria (laboratory or imaging)
Type III:
Pancreatic type pain only

Table 4. Modified Milwaukee Classification of Sphincter of Oddi dysfunction [8, 61, 62, 64-66].

As in biliary dyspepsia due to gallbladder dysfunction, patients with suspected SOD should undergo evaluation with serum liver and pancreas biochemical tests, abdominal ultrasound, and esophagogastroduodenoscopy to rule out underlying structural disease as a cause for their abdominal symptoms. Consideration should also be given to magnetic resonance cholangio-pancreatography (MRCP) to eliminate structural lesions such as stones, strictures and tumors. Dysfunction potentially might affect either or both segments of the sphincter of Oddi: biliary versus pancreatic sphincters or both (e.g.; occurring simultaneously).

a. Functional Biliary Sphincter of Oddi Disorder

Type I manifest biliary pain; abnormal liver biochemistries (elevated aminotransferases, alkaline phosphatase and/or bilirubin) >2 times normal on two or more occasions; plus a dilated common bile duct > 8mm on abdominal ultrasound. Most will exhibit biliary SO dysfunction on formal manometry. They are considered to have stenosis of the sphincter causing structural outflow obstruction.

Type II patients with biliary sphincter dysfunction experience the biliary-type pain plus exhibit one of either the laboratory or the imaging abnormalities.

Type III patients only complain of the pain. There are no laboratory or imaging abnormalities

b. Functional Pancreatic Sphincter of Oddi Disorder [65, 66]

Pancreatic-type SOD encompasses patients with pancreatic-type pain, elevated serum amylase or lipase plus pancreatic duct dilation.

Type I has pain, lipase elevation and pancreatic duct dilation

Type II has pain plus either lipase elevation or pancreatic duct dilation.

Type III has only pancreatic-type pain.

Investigations

1. ERCP Manometry.

The "gold" standard to diagnose SOD is sphincter of Oddi manometry. This entails endoscopic retrograde cholangiopancreatography (ERCP) allowing passage of a manometric catheter through the duct and measurement of basal sphincter pressures on slow withdrawal of the catheter. A basal sphincter pressure of greater than or equal to 40 mmHg is used to diagnose SOD [67]. Manometry is abnormal in 65-100% with type I, 50-65% with type II, and falls to 12-60% of biliary type III SOD patients [65, 67, 68]. Positive manometric findings, based on type, are similar in both types of sphincter dysfunction. The distinction between types I, II, and III SOD, however, is important as it may predict a favorable response to endoscopic sphincterotomy and thus, guide further management. The algorithm for diagnosing and treating functional biliary sphincter of Oddi dysfunction is outlined in Figure 4.

2. Non-invasive Methods

Additional non-invasive methods for diagnosing SOD have been studied, given the inherent risk of complications in sphincter of Oddi manometry, particularly precipitating pancreatitis, and the generally poor outcomes especially in patients with biliary type III SOD [69].

a. Ultrasonographic measurement of duct diameter

The common bile duct normally has a diameter of 6mm or less in healthy individuals whose gallbladders are intact. Above 8mm indicates biliary obstruction. This value becomes somewhat obscure following cholecystectomy, a situation in which dilation occurs to 10mm even in those without symptoms [70]. Adding a fatty meal to release CCK seeks to show duct dilation to indicate SO dysfunction but its diagnostic usefulness is limited.

b. Magnetic resonance pancreatography (MRCP)

Administration of the hormone secretin increases pancreatic exocrine secretion [71]. In suspected SOD involving the pancreas, secretin improves MRCP visualization of the pancreatic ducts to eliminate structural disease and elicits duct dilation [72]. Overall, secretin-stimulated magnetic resonance cholangiopancreatography (ss-MRCP) is not sensitive in predicting abnormal manometry results in patients with suspected SOD type III, though somewhat accurate in predicting results in patients with SOD type II (73%) [73].

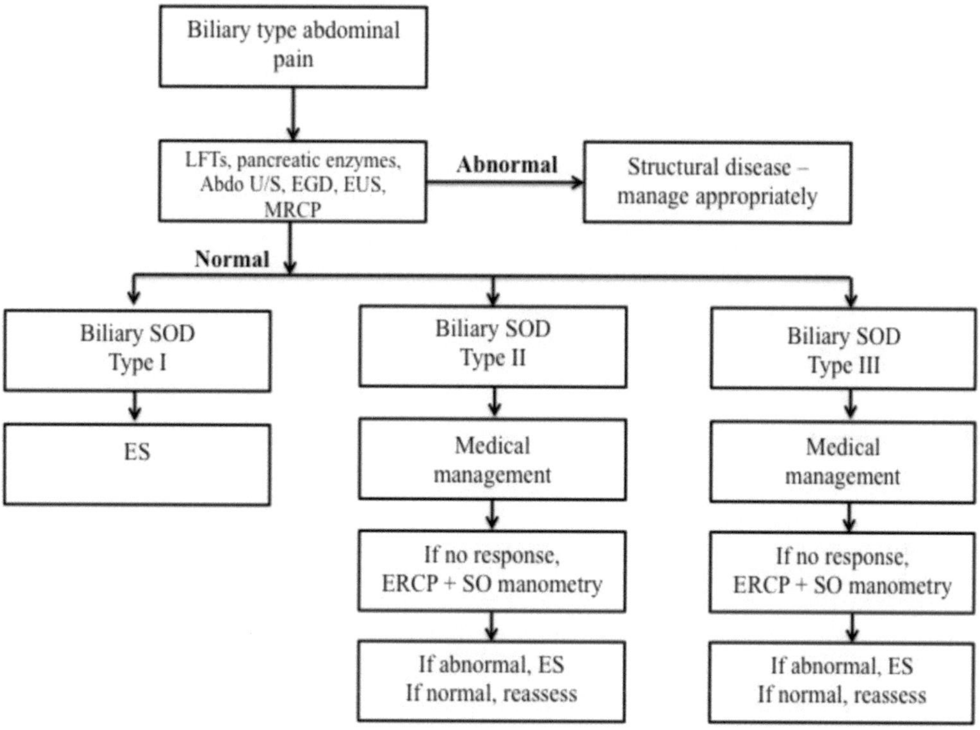

Figure 4. Algorithm for the diagnostic workup and management of sphincter of Oddi disorder (SOD) [8] Patients with biliary type pain should initially undergo non-invasive investigations including relevant laboratory work and an abdominal ultrasound. An endogastroduodenoscopy (EGD), endoscopic ultrasound (EUS) and a magnetic resonance cholangiopancreatography (MRCP) should then be performed. Any structural abnormalities detected should be treated by medical, endoscopic or surgical management. SOD should be classified as Type I, Type II and Type III according to the Milwaukee classification described in the text,. Patients with Type I disease will benefit from an endoscopic sphincterotomy (ES). Otherwise first line management should be medical. If there is no response, an ERCP with sphincter of Oddi manometry (SO manometry) can be performed. If manometry is abnormal, ES is indicated. If normal, alternative medical therapies can be attempted.

c. Endosonography

Endoscopic ultrasound (EUS) generally has a low yield in diagnosing abnormalities in the context of a normal upper endoscopy and imaging studies in patients with SOD Type III [72, 74]. Only 8% of patients with suspected SOD Type III (normal endoscopy and standard imaging studies) have any pathology at EUS [74].

d. Hepatobiliary scintigraphy [10]

Nuclear medicine scanning of the biliary tract (choledochoscintigraphy) uses 99mTc HIDA as the radiopharmaceutical to measure biliary emptying: the transit time from the liver to the duodenum. Prolonged duodenal arrival reflects SO dysfunction [75]. Specificity approaches 90% but reported sensitivities are variable [76]. Although lacking controlled studies, choledochoscintigraphy is a reasonable non-invasive test before embarking on an intrusive approach with ERCP-manometry.

e. Morphine-prostigmine provocation (Nardi) test

The Nardi test assesses the response to an injection of morphine and prostigmine to provoke biliary sphincter spasm and stimulate pancreatic enzyme secretion. A positive test should elicit typical symptoms and/or increase in serum activities of pancreatic and/or liver enzymes. This provocative test is not specific or sensitive: 60% of normal individuals and others with IBS have a positive test [77]. Sphincterotomy decreases the pain and enzymatic response (amylase and lipase) to such provocation in only about 50% of individuals [78].

6. Management

a. Functional Gallbladder Disorder

Medical

The medical options for management of functional biliary disorders are quite limited. The spice turmeric (Curcuma longa) modulates multiple cell signalling pathways and is a putative therapy for inflammatory bowel disease [79]. In patients with biliary dyspepsia, the extracts of Curcuma seem to reduce abdominal pain at least during the first week of treatment [80]. Oddly, curcumin increases gallbladder contraction. Tenoten, an anxiolytic, appeared to decrease the pain syndrome, burning and belching, and increase gallbladder contraction in a small Russian study assessing patients with biliary dyskinesia and personality disorders [81]. Such reports have marked limitations including small patient numbers and unclear diagnostic criteria for biliary dyspepsia. As such, further studies are needed to clarify any role for medical therapy in biliary dyskinesia, including use of agents like tricyclic antidepressants that help visceral hypersensitivity.

Surgical

Although there may be a rising tide of cholecystectomies being performed for biliary dyskinesia, most reports touting efficacy are retrospective reviews with small sample sizes and lack appropriate non-operative controls. One meta-analysis supported the notion of surgery in adults that provided 98% symptomatic relief compared to 32% with non-operative management [59]. Although the success rate in pediatric patients may reach 80% in some reports, a retrospective assessment of outcomes indicated no difference over a 2 year follow up: three-quarters of both the surgical and non-surgical groups improved [82]. Further, gallbladder emptying assessed by CCK-cholescintigraphy may not be a sensitive test that predicts a benefit from cholecystectomy [83]. Certainly cholecystectomy for dyspeptic complaints of gassiness, bloating, indigestion and fatty food intolerance is disappointing [84]. Despite the Rome III consensus [8], the literature does not yet support cholecystectomy being done routinely for biliary dyspepsia.

b. Functional Sphincter of Oddi Disorder

The aim in patients with SOD is to reduce the resistance caused by the sphincter of Oddi to the flow of bile and/or pancreatic juice [3]. This can be achieved by medical, endoscopic or surgical methods.

Medical

Medical management of sphincter of Oddi dysfunction is also unclear. Therapy has been primarily focused on the use of smooth muscle relaxants. Nifedipine, a calcium channel antagonist, has previously been studied with conflicting results in the treatment of sphincter of Oddi dysfunction. Nifedipine 20mg can significantly decrease the basal pressure in the sphincter of Oddi and also reduce the amplitude, duration and frequency of phasic contractions [85]. This effect is not seen at lower doses of nifedipine; unfortunately, hypotension is a common side effect at the higher dose. Nevertheless, nifedipine use over 3 months decreases pain, especially in patients with predominant antegrade propagation of phasic contractions [86]. Once treatment ceases, the effect becomes lost in a week [86]. Nicardipine also appears to have a similar effect on the sphincter of Oddi with a decrease in basal and phasic pressures following a single infusion [87].

Trimebutine (a spasmolytic), sublingual nitrates or a combination of both agents provides complete or partial relief of pain in most cases (64-71%) [88, 89]. All such studies however are limited by small patient numbers.

Several other medications such as anticholinergics (e.g.; hyoscine butylbromide), antispasmodics (e.g.; tiropramide), opioid antagonists (e.g.; naloxone), alpha-2 adrenergic agonists (e.g.; clonidine), and even corticosteroids may have a potential benefit in managing sphincter of Oddi dysfunction or functional gallbladder disorder [90]. Nevertheless, reports are limited in quality; well-done clinical trials are warranted.

Endoscopic Therapy

The goal of endoscopic therapy is to disable the dysfunctional sphincter through various methods. Botulinum toxin, a neurotoxin, when injected directly into the ampulla of Vater at endoscopy, improves symptoms in 44% of SOD patients for 6 to 12 weeks after the treatment [91]. Unfortunately, repeated injections of botulinum toxin may be associated with antibody formation and a subsequent reduced efficacy [90]. Hence, rather than being used to treat sphincter of Oddi dysfunction, botulinum toxin injections appear more helpful in directing further therapy, predicting the success of endoscopic sphincterotomy for pain relief [90, 91].

Endoscopic sphincterotomy (ES) is the current treatment for SOD Type I. At ERCP, deep cannulation of the bile (or pancreatic) duct allows electrocautery to sever the biliary or the pancreatic segment of the sphincter of Oddi. Pain relief after an ES is 90-95% in Type I patients, 85% in Type II patients with an abnormal sphincter of Oddi manometry and 55-60% in Type III patients with an abnormal manometry [92, 93]. Conversely, in patients with a normal manometry, the relief rates are much reduced: 35% for Type II and $<20\%$ in Type III patients, respectively [92, 93]. Complications from this procedure are mostly due to pancreatitis, which can be seen in up to 20% of patients [94]. ES as an indication of SOD results in a 2-5 fold increase in complications compared to the risk when performing this procedure for ductal stones [95, 96]. Placing a temporary stent in the pancreatic duct helps lessen such complications.

Surgical

Surgical options include transduodenal biliary sphincteroplasty with a transampullary septoplasty [97]. Due to the advances in endoscopic techniques, surgery is generally reserved for patients who experience restenosis or when endoscopy is not available [97]. Endoscopy is preferred with lower cost, morbidity and mortality compared to surgical procedures.

7. Summary

Functional gallbladder disease and sphincter of Oddi disorders can be quite frustrating for the patient as well as the physician, in terms of arriving at a diagnosis and effective therapeutic options. Initially, non-invasive investigations should be performed. Further, sphincter of Oddi manometry requires specialized endoscopic equipment as well as physician expertise. Unfortunately, this is not readily available in many centers. Perhaps with the procurement of these resources in the future, physicians may be able to predict which patients with SOD will benefit from endoscopic or surgical therapy. In terms of management, medical therapies should be tried as first line. Further, surgical and endoscopic management in type II and type III SOD should be initiated with caution. The suggested algorithm should assist the investigation and management of these patients (Figure 3 and 4).

Author details

Meena Mathivanan, Liisa Meddings and Eldon A. Shaffer*

*Address all correspondence to: shaffer@ucalgary.ca

Division of Gastroenterology, University of Calgary, Calgary, Alberta, Canada

References

[1] DiBaise JK. Evaluation and management of functional biliary pain in patients with an intact gallbladder. Expert Rev Gastroenterol Hepatol. 2009;3:305-313.

[2] Gracie WA, Ransohoff DF. The natural history of silent gallstones. The innocent gallstones are not a myth. New Engl J Med. 1982;307:798–800.

[3] Kraag N, Thijs C, Knipschild P. Dyspepsia—how noisy are gallstones? A meta-analysis of biliary pain, dyspepsia symptoms, and food. Scand J Gastroenterol. 1995;30:411–21.

[4] Mertens MC, Roukema JA, Scholtes VPW, De Vries J. Risk assessment in cholelithiasis: Is cholecystectomy always to be preferred? Gastrointest Surg. 2010;14:1271–1279.

[5] Festi D, Reggiani ML, Attili AF, Loria P, Pazzi P, Scaioli E, Capodiscasa S, Romano F, Roda E, Colecchia A. Natural history of gallstone disease: Expectant management or active treatment? Results from a population-based cohort study. J Gastroenterol Hepatol. 2010;25:719-724.

[6] Thistle JL, Longstreth GF, Romero Y, Arora AS, Simonson JA, Diehl NN, Harmsen WS, Zinsmeister AR. Factors That Predict Relief From Upper Abdominal Pain After Cholecystectomy. Clin Gastroenterol Hepatol. 2011;9: 891-6.

[7] Kirk G, Kennedy R, McKie L, Diamond T, Clements B. Preoperative symptoms of irritable bowel syndrome predict poor outcome after laparoscopic cholecystectomy. Surg Endosc. 2011, 25: 3379-3384.

[8] Behar J, Corazziari E, Guelrud M, Hogan W, Sherman S, Toouli J. Functional gallbladder and sphincter of oddi disorders. Gastroenterology. 2006;130:1498-1509.

[9] Hansel SL, DiBaise JK. Functional gallbladder disorder: Gallbladder dyskinesia. Gastroenterol Clin N Am. 2010;39:369-379.

[10] Shaffer, E. Acalculous biliary pain: new concepts for an old entity. Dig Liver Dis. 2003;35 (Suppl 3):S20-5.

[11] Varadarajulu S, Hawes R. Key issues in sphincter of Oddi dysfunction. Gastrointest Endosc Clin N Am. 2003;13:671-94.

[12] Oustamaanolakis P, Tack J. Dyspepsia: Organic versus functional. J Clin Gastroenterol. 2012;46:175-190.

[13] Agreus L. Natural history of dyspepsia. Gut. 2002; 50:2-9.

[14] Peery AF, Dellon ES, Lund J, Crockett SD, McGowan CE, Bulsiewicz WJ, Gangarosa LM, Thiny MT, Stizenberg K, Morgan DR, Ringel Y, Kim HP, Dibonaventura MD, Carroll CF, Allen JK, Cook SF, Sandler RS, Kappelman MD, Shaheen NJ. Burden of Gastrointestinal Disease in the United States: 2012 Update. Gastroenterology. 2012;143: 1179-1187.

[15] GREPCO (The Rome group for epidemiology and prevention of cholelithiasis). The epidemiology of gallstone disease in Rome, Italy. I. Prevalence data in men. Hepatology 1988;8:904–6.

[16] GREPCO (Rome group for epidemiology and prevention of cholelithiasis). Prevalence of gallstone disease in an Italian adult female population. Am J Epidemiol. 1984:119:796–805.

[17] Johanning JM, Gruenberg JC. The changing face of cholecystectomy. Am Surg. 1998;64: 643-7.

[18] Bielefeldt K. The rising tide of cholecystectomy for biliary dyskinesia. Aliment Pharmacol and Ther. 2013;37: 98-106.

[19] Raptopoulos V, Compton CC, Doherty P, Smith EH, D'Orsi CJ, Patwardhan NA, Goldberg R. Chronic acalculous gallbladder disease: multiimaging evaluation with clinical-pathologic correlation. Am J Roentgenol. 1986;147: 721–4.

[20] Chen PF, Nimeri A, Pham QH, Yuh JN, Gusz JR, Chung RS. The clinical diagnosis of chronic acalculous cholecystitis. Surgery. 2001; 130: 578–81.

[21] Patel NA, Lamb JJ, Hogle NJ, Fowler DL. Therapeutic efficacy of laparoscopic cholecystectomy in the treatment of biliary dyskinesia. Am J Surg. 2004;187:209–12.

[22] Joseph S, Moore BT, Sorensen GB, Earley JW, Tang F, Jones P, Brown KM. Single-incision laparoscopic cholecystectomy: a comparison with the gold standard. Surg Endosc. 2011; 25: 3008–15.

[23] St Peter SD, Keckler SJ, Nair A, Andrews WS, Sharp RJ, Snyder CL, Ostlie DJ, Holcomb GW. Laparoscopic cholecystectomy in the pediatric population. J Laparoendosc Adv Surg Tech A. 2008; 18:127–30.

[24] Al-Homaidhi HS, Sukerek H, Klein M, Tolia V. Biliary dyskinesia in children. Pediatr Surg Int. 2002;18:357–60.

[25] Hofeldt M, Richmond B, Huffman K, Nestor J, Maxwell D. Laparoscopic cholecystectomy for treatment of biliary dyskinesia is safe and effective in the pediatric population. Am Surg. 2008; 74: 1069–72.

[26] Kaye AJ, Jatla M, Mattei P, Kelly J, Nance ML. Use of laparoscopic cholecystectomy for biliary dyskinesia in the child. J Pediatr Surg. 2008; 43: 1057–9.

[27] Drossman DA, Li Z, Andruzzi E, Temple RD, Talley NJ, Thompson WG, Whitehead WE, Janssens J, Funch-Jensen P, Corazziari E et al. U.S. householder survey of functional gastrointestinal disorders. Prevalence, sociodemography, and health impact. Dig Dis Sci. 1993;38: 1569-80.

[28] Bar-Meir S, Halpern Z, Bardan E, Gilat T. Frequency of papillary dysfunction among cholecystectomized patients. Hepatology. 1984;4:328–330.

[29] Shaffer EA. Gallbladder motility in health disease. In: La Russo NF, editor, Gastroenterology and hepatology: the comprehensive visual reference volume, Gallbladder and bile ducts. Essential atlas of gastroenterology and hepatology for primary care, Philadelphia: Current Medicine Inc.; 1997, pp. 1–33, chapter 5.

[30] Cervero F, Laird JMA. From acute to chronic pain. Mechanisms and hypothesis. Prog Brain Res.1996;110:3–15.

[31] Mayer EA, Gebhart GF. Basic and clinical aspects of visceral hyperalgesia. Gastroenterology. 1994;107:271–93.

[32] Evans PR, Bak Y-T, Dowsett JF, Smith RC, Kellow JE. Small bowel dysmotility in patients with post-cholecystectomy sphincter of Oddi dysfunction. Dig Dis Sci. 1997;42:1507-12.

[33] Francis G, Baillie J. Gallbladder Dyskinesia: Fact or Fiction? Curr Gastroenterol Rep. 2011;13:188-192.

[34] Stinton L, Shaffer EA. Epidemiology of Gallbladder Disease: Cholelithiasis and Cancer. Gut and Liver. 2012; 6(2): 172-187.

[35] Pomeranz IS, Shaffer EA. Abnormal gallbladder emptying in a subgroup of patients with gallstones. Gastroenterology. 1985;91: 787-91.

[36] Xu QW, Shaffer EA. The potential site of impaired gallbladder contractility in an animal model of cholesterol gallstone disease. Gastroenterology. 1996; 110:251 257.

[37] Amaral J, Xiao ZL, Chen Q, Yu P, Biancani P, Behar J. Gallbladder muscle dysfunction in patients with chronic acalculous disease. Gastroenterology. 2001;120:506-511.

[38] Velanovich V. Biliary dyskinesia and biliary crystals: A prospective study. Am Surg. 1997;63:69-74.

[39] Westlake P, Hershfield NB, Kelly JK, Kloiber R, Lui R, Sutherland LR, Shaffer EA. Chronic right upper quadrant pain without gallstones: Does HIDA scan predict outcome after cholecystectomy? Am J Gastroenterology. 1991;86:375-376.

[40] Vassiliou MC, Laycock WS. Biliary dyskinesia. Surg Clin North Am. 2008; 88: 1253-1272.

[41] Marzio L. Factors affecting gallbladder motility: drugs. Dig Liver Dis. 2003;35:S17-9.

[42] Moriarty KJ, Dawson AM. Functional abdominal pain: further evidence that the whole gut is affected. Br Med J. 1982;284:1670-2.

[43] Evans PR, Dowsett JF, Bak YT, Chan YK, Kellow JE. Abnormal sphincter of Oddi response to cholecystokinin in postcholecystectomy syndrome patients with irritable bowel syndrome. The irritable sphincter. Dig Dis Sci. 1995;40:1149-56.

[44] Kamath PS, Gaisano HY, Phillips SF, Miller LJ, Charboneau JW, Brown ML, Zinsmeister AR. Abnormal gallbladder motility in irritable bowel syndrome: evidence for target-organ defect. Am J Physiol. 1991:260: G815-9.

[45] Sood GK, Baijal SS, Lahoti D, Broor SL. Abnormal gallbladder function in patients with irritable bowel syndrome. Am J Gastroenterol. 1993;88:1387-90.

[46] Kellow JE. Sphincter of Oddi dysfunction type III: another manifestation of visceral hyperalgesia? Gastroenterology. 1999:116:996-1000.

[47] Desautels SG, Slivka A, Huston WR, Chun A, Mitrani C, DiLorenzo C, Wald A. Postcholecystectomy pain syndrome; pathophysiology of abdominal pain in sphincter of Oddi type III. Gastroenterology. 1999; 116 (4): 900–905.

[48] Kaess H, Kellermann M, Castro A. Food intolerance in duodenal ulcer patients, non ulcer dyspeptic patients and health subjects. A prospective study. Klin Wochenschr 1998;66:208-211.

[49] Mullan A, Kavanagh P, O'Mahony P, Joy T, Gleeson F, Gibney MJ. Food and nutrient intakes and eating patterns in functional and organic dyspepsia. Eur J Clin Nutr. 1994;48:97-105.

[50] Pilichiwicz, AN, Feltrin KL, Horowitz M, Holtmann G, Wishart JM, Jones KL, Talley NJ, Feinle-Bisset C. Functional dyspepsia is associated with a greater symptomatic response to fat but not carbohydrate, increased fasting and postprandial CCK, and diminished PYY. Am J Gastroenterol. 2008;103:2613-23.

[51] Pilichiewicz AN, Horowitz M, Holtmann GJ, Talley NJ, Feinle-Bisset C. Relationship between symptoms and dietary patterns in patients with functional dyspepsia. Clin Gastroenterol and Hepatol. 2009;7:317-322.

[52] Festi D, Dormi A, Capodicasa S, Staniscia T, Attili AF, Loria P, Pazzi P, Mazzella G, Sama C, Roda E, Colecchia A. Incidence of gallstone disease in Italy: results from a multicenter, population-based Italian study (the MICOL project). World J Gastroenterol. 2008;14:5282–9.

[53] Shaffer, EA. Gallstone Disease: From dyspepsia to biliary complications. J Clin Outcomes Manag. 2009;16: 37-48.

[54] Dill JE, Hill S, Callis J, Berkhouse L, Evans P, Martin D, Palmer ST. Combined endoscopic ultrasound and stimulated biliary drainage in cholecystitis and microlithiasis – diagnoses and outcomes. Endoscopy. 1995;27:424-7.

[55] Dahan P, Andant C, Levy P, Amouyal P, Amouyal G, Dumont M, Erlinger S, Sauvanet A, Belghiti J, Zins M, Vilgrain V, Bernades P. Prospective evaluation of endoscopic ultrasonography and microscopic examination of duodenal bile in the diagnosis of cholecystolithiasis in 45 patients with normal conventional ultrasonography. Gut. 1996;38:277-281.

[56] Dauer M, Lammert F. Mandatory and optional function tests for biliary disorders. Best Pract Res Clin Gastroenterol. 2009;23(3): 441-451.

[57] DiBaise JK, Richmond BK, Ziessman HA, Everson GT, Fanelli RD, Maurer AH, Ouyang A, Shamamian P, Simons RJ, Wall LA, Weida TJ, Tulchinsky M. Cholecystokinin-cholescintigraphy in adults: consensus recommendations of an interdisciplinary panel. Clin Nucl Med. 2012;37: 63–70.

[58] DiBaise JK, Richmond BK, Ziessman HH, Everson GT, Maurer A, Ouyang A, Shamamian P, Simons RJ, Wall LA, Weida TJ, Tulchinsky M. Cholecystokinin-cholescintig-

raphy in adults: consensus recommendations of an interdisciplinary panel. Clin Gastroenterol Hepatol. 2011;9: 376–84.

[59] Ponsky TA, DeSagun R, Brody F. Surgical therapy for biliary dyskinesia: a meta-analysis and review of the literature. J Laparoendosc Adv Surg Tech A. 2005;15: 439-442.

[60] Irshad A, Ackerman SJ, Spicer K, Baker N, Campbell A, Anis M, Shazly M. Ultrasound evaluation of gallbladder dyskinesia: Comparison of scintigraphy and dynamic 3D and 4D ultrasound techniques. AJR Am J Roentgenol. 2011;197: 1103-1110.

[61] Smythe A, Majeed AW, Fitzhenry M, Johnson AG. A requiem for the cholecystokinin provocation test? Gut. 1998;43:571-4.

[62] Hogan WJ, Geenen JE. Biliary dyskinesia. Endoscopy. 1988;20: 179-183.

[63] Geenen JE, Hogan WJ, Dodds WJ, Toouli J, Venu RP. The efficacy of endoscopic sphincterotomy after cholecystectomy in patients with sphincter-of-Oddi dysfunction. N Engl J Med. 1989; 320: 82-7.

[64] Baillie J. Sphinter of Oddi dysfunction: overdue for an overhaul. Am J Gastroenterol. 2005;100:1217-20.

[65] Petersen BT. Sphincter of Oddi dysfunction, part 2: evidence- based review of the presentations, with "objective" pancreatic findings (types I and II) and of presumptive type III. Gastrointest Endosc. 2004;59:670-686.

[66] Elta GH. Sphincter of Oddi dysfunction and bile duct microlithiasis in acute idiopathic pancreatitis. World J Gastroenterol. 2008;14:1023-6.

[67] Pfau PR, Banerjee S, Barth BA, Desilets DJ, Kaul V, Kethu SR, Pedrosa MC, Pleskow DK, Tokar J, Varadarajulu S, Wang A, Song LM, Rodriguez SA. Sphincter of Oddi manometry. Gastrointest Endosc. 2011;74:1175-80.

[68] Sherman S, Troiano FP, Hawes RH, O'Connor KW, Lehman GA. Frequency of abnormal sphincter of Oddi manometry compared with the clinical suspicion of sphincter of Oddi dysfunction. Am J Gastroenterol. 1991;86:586-90.

[69] Sgouros SN, Pereira SP. Systematic review: sphincter of Oddi dysfunction - non-invasive diagnostic methods and long-term outcome after endoscopic sphincterotomy. Aliment Pharmacol Ther. 2006;24(2): 237-246.

[70] Senturk S, Miroglu TC, Bilici A, Gumus H, Tekin RC, Ekici F, Tekbas G. Diameters of the common bile duct in adults and postcholecystectomy patients: a study with 64-slice CT. Eur J Radiol. 2012;81:39-42.

[71] Carr-Locke DL, Gregg JA, Chey WY. Effects of exogenous secretin on pancreatic and biliary ductal and sphincteric pressures in man demonstrated by endoscopic manometry and correlation with plasma secretin levels. Dig Dis Sci. 1985;30:909-17.

[72] Aisen AM, Sherman S, Jennings SG, Fogel EL, Li T, Cheng CL, Devereaux BM, McHenry L, Watkins JL, Lehman GA. Comparison of secretin-stimulated magnetic resonance pancreatography and manometry results in patients with suspected sphincter of oddi dysfunction. Acad Radiol. 2008;15(5): 601-609.

[73] Pereira SP, Gillams A, Sgouros SN, Webster GJ, Hatfield AR. Prospective comparison of secretin-stimulated magnetic resonance cholangiopancreatograpy with manometry in the diagnosis of sphincter of Oddi dysfunction types II and III. Gut. 2007;56(6): 809-813.

[74] Siddiqui AA, Tholey D, Kedika R, Loren DE, Kowalski TE, Eloubeidi MA. Low but significant yield of endosonography in patients with suspected Sphincter of Oddi Dysfunction Type III with normal imaging studies. J Gastrointestin Liver Dis. 2012; 21: 271-275.

[75] Shaffer EA, Hershfield NB, Logan K, Kloiber R. Cholescintigraphic detection of functional obstruction of the sphincter of Oddi. Effect of papillotomy. Gastroenterology. 1986;90:728–33.

[76] Corazziari E, Cicala M, Scopinaro F, Schillaci O, Habib IF, Pallotta N. Scintigraphic assessment of SO dysfunction. Gut. 2003;52:1655-6.

[77] Steinberg WM, Salvato RF, Toskes PP. The morphine-prostigmin provocative test – is it useful for making clinical decisions? Gastroenterology. 1980; 78:728-31.

[78] Lobo DN, Takhar AS, Thaper A, Dube MG, Rowlands BJ. The morphine-prostigmine provocation (Nardi) test for sphincter of Oddi dysfunction: results in healthy volunteers and in patients before and after transduodenal sphincteroplasty and transampullary septectomy. Gut. 2007;56: 1472-73.

[79] Gupta SC, Patchva S, Aggarwal BB. Therapeutic roles of curcumin: lessons learned from clinical trials. AAPS J. 2013:15:195-218.

[80] Niederau C, Gopfert E. The effect of chelidonium – and turmeric root extract on upper abdominal pain due to functional disorders of the biliary system. Results from a placebo-controlled double-blind study. Med Klin. 1999; 94:425-30.

[81] Simanenkov VI, Poroshina EG, Tikhonov SV. The use of tenoten preparation in complex therapy of hypomotoric biliary dyskinesia. Bull Exp Biol Med. 2009;148: 349-350.

[82] Scott Nelson R, Kolts R, Park R, Heikenen J. A comparison of cholecystectomy and observation in children with biliary dyskinesia. J Pediatr Surg. 2006, 41:1894-98.

[83] DiBaise JK, Oleynikov D. Does gallbladder ejection fraction predict outcome after cholecystectomy for suspected chronic acalculous gallbladder dysfunction? A systematic review. Am J Gastroenterol. 2003;98:2605-11.

[84] Fenster LF, Lonborg R, Thirlby RC, Traverso LW. What symptoms does cholecystectomy cure? Insights from an outcome measurement project and review of literature. Am J Surg. 1995;169: 533-38.

[85] Guelrud M, Mendoza S, Rossiter G, Ramirez L, Barkin J. Effect of nifedipine on sphincter of Oddi motor activity: studies in healthy volunteers and patients with biliary dyskinesia. Gastroenterology. 1988;95:1050-55.

[86] Khuroo, MS, Zargar, SA & Yattoo, GN. Efficacy of nifedipine therapy in patients with sphincter of Oddi dysfunction: a prospective, double-blind, randomized, placebo-controlled, cross over trial. Br J Clin Pharmacol. 1992; 33:477–85.

[87] Fullarton GM, Falconer S, Campbell A, Murray WR. Controlled study of the effect of nicardipine and ceruletide on the sphincter of Oddi. Gut. 1992;33: 550-53.

[88] Vitton V, Ezzedine S, Gonzalez JM, Gasmi M, Grimaud J, Barthet M. Medical treatment for sphincter of oddi dysfunction: can it replace endoscopic sphincterotomy? World J Gastroenterol. 2012;18: 1610-5.

[89] Vitton V, Delpy R, Gasmi M, Lesavre N, Abou-Berdugo E, Desjeux A, Grimaud J, Barthet M. Is endoscopic sphincterotomy avoidable in patients with sphincter of Oddi dysfunction? Eur J Gastroenterol Hepatol. 2008;20:15-21.

[90] Craig A, Toouli J. Sphincter of Oddi dysfunction: is there a role for medical therapy? Curr Gastroenterol Rep. 2002;4: 172-6.

[91] Murray WR. Botulinum toxin-induced relaxation of the sphincter of Oddi may select patients with acalculous biliary pain who will benefit from cholecystectomy. Surg Endosc. 2011;25: 813-16.

[92] Fullarton GM, Murray WR. Evaluation of endoscopic sphincterotomy in sphincter of Oddi dysfunction. Endoscopy. 1992;24:199-202.

[93] Sugawa C, Park DH, Lucas CE, Higuchi D, Ukawa K. Endoscopic sphincterotomy for stenosis of the sphincter of Oddi. Surg Endosc. 2001;15:1004-7.

[94] Sherman S. What is the role of ERCP in the setting of abdominal pain of pancreatic or biliary origin (suspected sphincter of Oddi dysfunction)? Gastrointest Endosc. 2002;56:S258-S266.

[95] Freeman ML, Nelson DB, Sherman S, Haber GB, Herman ME, Dorsher PJ, Moore JP, Fennerty MB, Ryan ME, Shaw MJ, Lande JD, Pheley AM. Complications of endoscopic biliary sphinterotomy. N Engl J Med. 1996;26:908-18.

[96] Sherman S, Ruffolo TA, Hawes RH, Lehman GA. Complications of endoscopic sphincterotomy. A prospective series with emphasis on the increased risk associated with sphincter of Oddi dysfunction and nondilated bile ducts. Gastroenterology. 1991;101:1068-75.

[97] Sherman S, Lehman G. Sphincter of Oddi dysfunction: diagnosis and treatment. JOP. 2001;2:382-400.

Chapter 8

Upper Gastrointestinal Symptoms and Cardiovascular Disease

Craig I. Coleman, Brendan L. Limone, Jeff R. Schein,
Winnie W. Nelson, Joyce C. LaMori,
Jeffrey Kluger and C. Michael White

Additional information is available at the end of the chapter

http://dx.doi.org/10.5772/56564

1. Introduction

Cardiovascular disease, primarily encompassing coronary heart disease, hypertensive heart disease, heart failure, and stroke, is the number one cause of death globally, with 17.3 million dying from such causes in 2008 and a projected 23.6 million dying from cardiovascular disease in 2030 [1]. Cardiovascular disease affects 1 in every 3 Americans, or an estimated 83.6 million people (myocardial infraction, 7.6 million; angina pectoris, 7.8 million; heart failure, 5.1 million; and stroke of any kind, 6.8 million; high blood pressure, 77.9 million) [2]. Heart disease and stroke results in over 500,000 and 160,000 deaths, respectively, each year in the United States; giving rise to an enormous annual economic burden exceeding $312 billion in both direct and indirect costs [1,2].

Upper gastrointestinal (or dyspeptic) symptoms, often sub-classified as ulcer-like (localized epigastric pain or nocturnal/fasting pain), gastroesophageal-like (heartburn or regurgitation) or dysmotility-like dyspepsia (postprandial fullness, early satiety, diffuse epigastric pain, belching or abdominal distention) are also highly prevalent worldwide with an average 3-month prevalence rate across an international sample of survey respondents of about 28%, but with higher rates in some countries such as the United States (41.8%) [3] and lower rates in others (Japan's rate=9.4%). Clinically-relevant upper gastrointestinal symptoms have been found to result in high healthcare utilization [4,5]; as noted in one study [4] which found 20% of affected patients visited a physician's office during the 3-months prior to being surveyed, 2% were hospitalized, nearly half used an over-the-counter medication and 27% were prescribed at least one medication to address their symptoms. Upper gastrointestinal symptoms have also been associated with significant costs due to lost work productivity [4,5], with those suffering symptoms having an 85% (95% confidence interval, 40%-145%) increased odds of work absenteeism [5], 27% reporting at least one day of reduced or no productivity over a 3-month period, and 89% of this subset of people reported more than one day affected [4]. In addition to these direct and indirect costs, increased intangible costs (pain and suffering) are also an important repercussion of upper gastrointestinal symptoms [6], with these symptoms shown to be associated with significantly impaired wellbeing and patients' ability to perform activities of daily life (subjects reporting relevant upper gastrointestinal symptoms had significantly worse Psychological General Well-Being Index (PGWBI) and Interference with Daily Life Index (IDLI) scores compared with those reporting no or non-relevant symptoms (PGWBI score 65.24 versus 77.91, $p<0.0001$; IDLI score 75.85 versus 98.57, $p<0.0001$). Both cardiovascular disease and upper gastrointestinal symptoms are common diagnoses in daily practice. According to the American Academy of Family Physicians, numerous diagnosis codes for both cardiovascular disease and upper gastrointestinal symptoms are among the most frequently billed for [7].

In addition, cardiovascular and upper gastrointestinal disorders are among the top 20 leading diagnoses for direct health expenditures in the United States [2]. In 2008, approximately $95.6 billion dollars were spent treating heart conditions and $27.2 billion were spent treating upper gastrointestinal disorders, making these two disease states the first and twelfth most costly diagnoses, respectively, for direct healthcare expenditures. Since cardiovascular disease and upper gastrointestinal symptoms are both common conditions, some overlap in the occurrence of these conditions would naturally be expected.

Diagnosis description	Diagnosis code (ICD-9-CM)
Cardiovascular disease	
Atrial fibrillation	427.31
Chronic ischemic heart disease, unspec.	414.9
Heart failure, congestive, unspec.	428.0
Hypertension, benign	401.1
Hypertension, unspecified	401.9
Chest pain, unspec.	786.50
Upper gastrointestinal symptoms	
Gastroenteritis, noninfectious, unspec.	558.9
Gastroesophageal reflux, no esophagitis	530.81
Nausea w/ vomiting	787.01

Table 1. International Classification of Diseases, Ninth Revision, Clinical Modification Codes for Cardiovascular Disease and Upper Gastrointestinal Symptoms Designated in the Top 100 According to the '*Family Practice Management Short List*' [reference 7]

http://dx.doi.org/10.5772/56564

Beyond both having relatively high frequencies in daily practice and large economic burdens, there are clinical data supporting the hypothesis that upper gastrointestinal symptoms are more prevalent in patients with cardiovascular disease. Previous studies have found upper gastrointestinal symptoms to occur as much as twice as often [8] in patients suffering from a cardiovascular disease [9-13], and moreover, some upper gastrointestinal disorder may increase patients' risk for cardiovascular disease [14-17].

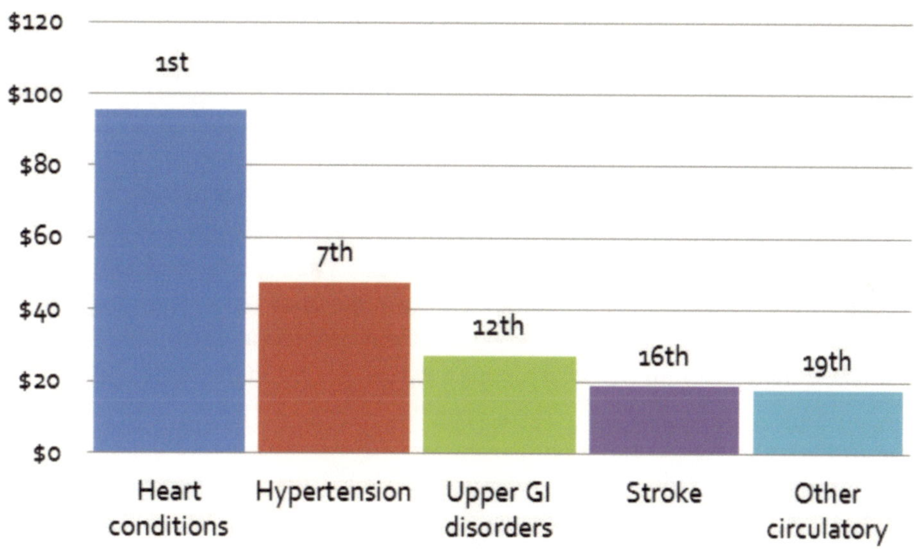

Figure 1. Cardiovascular Disease and Upper Gastrointestinal Symptoms on the List of 20 Leading Diagnoses for Direct Healthcare Expenditures (adapted from reference 2) Bars depicts the cost each diagnosis in 2008 US$, while the labels above the bars provides each diagnosis' ranking in direct healthcare expenditures.

The finding of higher prevalence rates of upper gastrointestinal symptoms in patients with cardiovascular disease may exist for a number of reasons. First, there are a host of mutual risk factors for developing both cardiovascular disease and upper gastrointestinal symptoms [18-37]. Next, patients experiencing both health problems often complain of similar or overlapping symptomatology, potentially resulting in the more frequent surveillance and diagnosis of both [38]. Related to this, some studies have suggested that common means of investigating upper gastrointestinal symptom origin can aggravate some cardiovascular diseases or induce cardiovascular symptoms [39,40]. Finally, polypharmacy with drugs used to manage cardiovascular diseases can cause upper gastrointestinal symptoms [8,41-46] resulting in decreased adherence to their medications, and a perhaps initiating a cycle of recurrence/worsening of cardiovascular disease. Moreover, some drugs to treat upper gastrointestinal symptoms may increase cardiovascular disease risk either directly or through drug-drug interactions.

The aim of this chapter is to provide a detailed discussion of the evidence suggesting and supporting an increased risk of upper gastrointestinal symptoms in populations suffering from cardiovascular disease.

2. Evidence supporting the link between cardiovascular disease and upper gastrointestinal symptoms

At least a half dozen published studies [8-13] have demonstrated a link between cardiovascular diseases and an increased risk of upper gastrointestinal symptoms. Three of these studies have assessed the association of upper gastrointestinal symptoms with general cardiovascular diagnosis. A recent study created two cohorts of patients derived from health insurance claims data from the Human Capital Management Services research database over a four year period (2001-2004)[9]. The cohorts were based upon the presence or absence of functional dyspepsia diagnosis codes, with the control cohort (n=83,450) being matched to the functional dyspepsia cohort (n=1,669) using a propensity score that included variables such as age, sex, marital status, salary, among others. This study demonstrated that employees with functional dyspepsia were 1.8-fold more likely to suffer from circulatory system disease (prevalence=39.19% in those with functional dyspepsia versus 22.37% in the control group; $p<0.05$).

Study, year (N=)	Study Description	Key Finding
Brook 2012 (N=275,875)	Retrospective database analysis of paid health insurance claims within the Human Capital Management Services research database (USA); 275,875 eligible employees, 1,669 with functional dyspepsia diagnosis codes	Higher prevalence of circulatory system disease in those with functional dyspepsia versus controls (ratio=1.8:1; prevalence=39.19% in those with functional dyspepsia versus 22.37% in the control group; p<0.05)
Stanghellini 1999 (N=5,581)	Respondents of the Domestic/International Gastroenterology Surveillance Study which surveyed urban, adult populations from 10 countries representing seven geographic areas (Canada, the USA, Switzerland, The Netherlands, Italy, Japan and the Nordic countries) using a study-specific symptom checklist; prevalence rate of upper gastrointestinal symptoms=28%	Higher odds of cardiovascular condition (OR=2.0), myocardial/endocardial/pericardial/valve condition (OR=2.7) or vascular (extracardiac) condition (OR=2.8) in patients with UGIS diagnosed by a doctor Higher odds of self-reported cardiovascular symptoms (OR=1.5), or myocardial/endocardial/pericardial/valve symptoms (OR=4.4) over previous three months in patients with UGIS
Wallander 2007 (N=17,949)	Analysis UK General Practice Research Database to identify patients with new onset dyspepsia in 1996; overall incidence=15.3	Higher odds of chest pain (OR: 2.4, 95%CI 2.1-2.7) or angina (OR=1.5, 95%CI=1.2-1.8) comorbidity in dyspepsia cohort in the year prior to index date than control cohort

http://dx.doi.org/10.5772/56564

Study, year (N=)	Study Description	Key Finding
	(95%CI 15.0-15.6) per 1000 person-years (n=6,913)	Higher odds of having first time diagnosis of chest pain (OR=2.3, 95%CI=2.0-2.8) or angina (OR=2.7, 95%CI=1.8-4.0) in dyspepsia group in the year after index date than in control cohort
Lohr 1986 (N=4,962)	Respondents completing a questionnaire enrolled in the Rand Health Insurance Experiment from six sites (Dayton, Ohio; Seattle, Washington; Fitchburg, Massachusetts; Franklin County, Massachusetts; Charleston, South Carolina; and Georgetown County, South Carolina); prevalence rate of ulcer-like symptoms per 100 (aged 18-61 years) men=3.8 and women=3.8	Congestive heart failure and angina were associated with a 3.6-fold ($p<0.001$) and 2.9-fold ($p<0.05$) higher odds of ulcer-like symptoms
LaMori 2012 (N=1,297)	Respondents to the 2009 National Health and Wellness Survey, a nationwide (USA) self-administered internet-based questionnaire; prevalence rate of dyspepsia=34%	Dyspepsia more likely among patients with higher stroke risk ($CHADS_2 \geq 2$, OR=1.15) Patients reporting dyspepsia in addition to AF had higher mean $CHADS_2$ scores (1.9 vs. 1.4, $p<0.05$)
Laliberte 2012 (N=413,168)	Retrospective database study of Thomson Reuters MarketScan data from 2005 and 2009 to quantify the incidence of dyspeptic events in patients with atrial fibrillation; median follow-up of 563 days	Incidence rate of dyspepsia was found to be 14.7 per 100-patients years
Pasini 1989 (N=NR)	Italian patients affected with congestive heart failure and ischemic heart disease studied to ascertain relation between dyspeptic syndrome and acute cardiac disorders	Data showed alterations of motility in esophagus, stomach, duodenum in every patient and lesions of gastric mucous membrane in more than half

AF=atrial fibrillation; FD=Functional dyspepsia; HLD=hyperlipidemia; HTN=hypertension; NA=not applicable; NR=not reported; OR=odds ratio; UK=United Kingdom; UGIS=upper gastrointestinal symptoms; USA=United States of America

Table 2. Studies Assessing Upper Gastrointestinal Symptoms in Patients with Cardiovascular Disease

A second study, the large Domestic/International Gastroenterology Surveillance Study [8] looked to investigate any association between upper gastrointestinal symptoms (gastroesophageal-, ulcer- or dysmotility-like) and lifestyle factors (including comorbidities) in a large sample of patients experiencing dyspepsia in the prior 3-months. A sample of urban, adult populations from seven geographic areas (Canada, United States, Switzerland, the Netherlands, Italy, Japan and the Nordic countries) was obtained by door-to-door or telephone recruitment. Subjects were divided into groups depending on whether gastrointestinal symptoms were reported and were analyzed for the association with comorbid conditions. In total, 5,581 subjects were recruited, with 1,566 (28%) reporting relevant upper gastrointestinal symptoms. In the previous three months, subjects reporting gastrointestinal symptoms self-reported more general cardiovascular (odds ratio= 1.5) or vascular myocardial/endocardial/pericardial and valve (odds ratio=4.4) symptoms or illnesses. Subjects with upper gastrointestinal symptoms also had increased prevalence of clinician-diagnosed cardiovascular (odds ratio=2.0) or myocardial/endocardial/pericardial and valve (odds ratio=2.7) conditions.

Two more large studies [10,11] have reported on a link between the prevalence of upper gastrointestinal symptoms with angina and chest pain. The first, a cross-sectional study of 6,913 patients aged 20-79 with new diagnoses of dyspepsia and 11,036 age- and sex-matched control patients from the United Kingdom-based General Practice Research Database, demonstrated dyspeptic patients are at increased odds of having a diagnosis for chest pain (odds ratio=2.4, 95% confidence interval=2.1-2.7) or angina (odds ratio=1.5, 95% confidence interval=1.2-1.8) within the previous year. In addition, dyspeptic patients are also more likely to receiving receive a first time diagnosis for chest pain (odds ratio=2.3, 95% confidence interval=2.0-2.8) or angina (odds ratio=2.7, 95% confidence interval=1.8-4.0) [10]. In an older study of 4,962 patients aged 18-61 who took part in the Rand Health Insurance Experiment, a decade-long randomized controlled trial of the effects of alternative methods of financing health care services, about 30% had one chronic illness, with an additional 16% having 2 or more. Ulcer-like symptoms, defined by a previous diagnosis along with taking antacids daily, frequent episodes of stomach pain relieved by milk, occurring one-half hour after eating or at night, was significantly associated with angina ($p<0.05$) and congestive heart failure ($p<0.001$) [11].

A single study sought to assess the prevalence of dyspepsia among patients with atrial fibrillation [12]. The population (n=1,297) included a nationwide sample of American adults (from the 2009 National Health and Wellness Survey) with atrial fibrillation divided into two groups: those reporting dyspepsia (defined as any of the following: ulcers, abdominal bloating, abdominal pain, gastroesophageal disease or heartburn) and those who did not. Of these atrial fibrillation patients, 41% reported a diagnosis of a gastrointestinal condition while 34% reported a diagnosis of dyspepsia. Patients with dyspepsia were associated with a significantly higher mean $CHADS_2$ score (1.9 vs. 1.4, $p<0.05$). Of note, while the $CHADS_2$ score was developed as a tool to determine atrial fibrillation patients' risk for stroke, in this case, it can also serve as a marker of the presence of cardiovascular diseases since 2 of 5 $CHADS_2$ criteria (eg, stroke and congestive heart failure) are in fact cardiovascular diseases and the remaining 3 criteria (eg, age, hypertension, diabetes) are potent risk factors for cardiovascular disease.

A retrospective database study sought to assess the risk of dyspepsia among patients with atrial fibrillation [13]. Analysis of insurance claims from the MarketScan® database from 2005-2009 was conducted. The population (n=413,168) included patients ≥18 years at the date of first atrial fibrillation diagnosis, with 180 days of continuous insurance coverage prior to the index atrial fibrillation diagnosis, and no gastrointestinal event within 180 days of the index atrial fibrillation diagnosis. The risk of dyspepsia was assessed with incidence rates (IRs; new dyspepsia case per patient years of observation). During a mean follow-up of 563 days, the IR

http://dx.doi.org/10.5772/56564

of dyspepsia for patients with atrial fibrillation was 14.7 events per 100 patient years. At baseline, 62% of patients (n=257,357) had at least one medication which may cause gastrointestinal tolerability issues. The authors conclude that atrial fibrillation was associated with a 40% risk of developing a gastrointestinal event, which was predominantly dyspepsia.

Finally in a small case series evaluating the relationship between dyspepsia and congestive heart disease or ischemic heart disease in Italian patients, data showed alterations of motility in the esophagus, stomach and duodenum in every cardiovascular disease patient evaluated and lesions of the gastric mucous membrane in more than half [14].

In addition to the aforementioned data suggesting upper gastrointestinal symptoms are more prevalent with patients with cardiovascular diseases; a body of literature suggesting upper gastrointestinal symptoms may in fact induce cardiovascular disease has begun to take shape [15-18]. In 2003, the first signal that gastro esophageal-like symptoms or disease could be linked to the development of atrial fibrillation was published [15]. Clinicians in Australia looked at 18 patients with concomitant diagnoses of lone paroxysmal atrial fibrillation and gastroesophageal reflux disease and noted that after treatment with a proton pump inhibitor to treat the upper gastrointestinal symptoms, 14 of 18 had a decrease or disappearance of at least one paroxysmal atrial fibrillation symptom.

Since that time, 3 observational studies [16-18] have more thoroughly evaluated this link. In a cohort study of 163,627 patients receiving care from the United States Army National Capitol Area Military Healthcare System between 2001 and 2007 (5% had atrial fibrillation and 29% had gastroesophageal-like symptoms), gastroesophageal symptoms were associated with an increased risk of atrial fibrillation, even after adjusting for age, sex, race and atherosclerotic risk factors (relative risk=1.19, 95% confidence interval=1.13-1.25) or further adjustment for ischemic heart disease, cardiomyopathy, atrial septal defect and being status post-cardiac bypass surgery (relative risk=1.08, 95% confidence interval=1.02-1.13) [16].

The second study [17] similarly sought to assess the relationship between gastroesophageal reflux disease and atrial fibrillation; and the researchers assessed the risk for atrial fibrillation over a follow-up period of greater than 11 years. A self-report survey was sent to 5,288 patients aged 25-74 over the 6 year period of 1988-1994. Of these patients, 741 developed atrial fibrillation. Contrary to the previous study, an inverse relationship with observed between gastroesophageal reflux disease symptoms and atrial fibrillation risk (hazard ratio=0.81, 95% confidence interval=0.68-0.96). However, the frequency of symptoms in those with gastroesophageal reflux (none, some, weekly, daily) was associated with an increased hazard of atrial fibrillation ($p<0.01$ for overall association); with daily symptoms associated with the highest hazard (hazard ratio=1.30, 95% Confidence interval=0.98-1.57) of developing atrial fibrillation compared to no gastroesophageal symptoms ($p=0.07$ unadjusted and $p>0.2$ after adjustment for confounders). The researchers cite an increase in medical attention in those experiencing gastroesophageal reflux as a possible explanation for the lack of association between the presence of symptoms and atrial fibrillation; hypothesizing that extra physician visits resulting from gastroesophageal symptoms resulted in early and more frequent identification and treatment of known atrial fibrillation risk factors, as well as a higher utilization of proton pump

Study, year (N=)	Study Description	Key Finding
Weigl 2003 (N=18)	Endoscopic reports of 640 Austrian patients searched for diagnosis of lone PAF and mention of reflux esophagitis; 18 patients invited to assess the effect of PPI therapy for GERD on paroxysmal AF-related symptoms	PPI therapy led to a decrease or disappearance of at least one PAF-related symptom in 14 of 18 patients.
Kunz 2009 (N=163,627)	Cross-sectional cohort study of adults in the United States Army National Capitol Area Military Healthcare System database; 7,992 patients with diagnosis of AF; 47,845 with diagnosis of GERD	GERD associated with increased risk of AF (RR=1.39, 95%CI=1.33-1.45; aRR=1.19, 95%CI=1.13-1.25#; aRR=1.08, 95%CI=1.02-1.13†)
Bunch 2009 (N=5,288)	Longitudinal survey study of Olmstead County, Minnesota residents to assess long-term risk of AF with symptomatic GERD; 2,577 (49%) reported GERD; 741 (14%) developed AF over 11.4 year follow-up period	The presence of GERD was associated with a decreased risk of AF (HR=0.81, 95%CI=0.68-0.96) The frequency of symptoms in those with GERD was associated with an increased hazard of AF ($p<0.01$); with daily symptoms associated with the highest risk (HR=1.30, 95% CI=0.98-1.57; p=0.07) compared to none.
Shimazu 2011 (N=188)	Cross-sectional survey study of Japanese patients completing screening questionnaire for GERD based upon frequency of 12 common symptoms to evaluate the relationship between AF and GERD; 46% with AF	AF was associated with prevalence of GERD (F-scale score≥8 points) ($p<0.001$ upon multivariate analysis). The dyspeptic sub-score (2.05±0.29 vs. 0.94±0.12, p =0.018) and the total F-scale score (3.98±0.51 vs. 2.12±0.21, p = 0.019) of AF patients were significantly greater than those in normal sinus rhythm.

*Widely used questionnaire in Japan to screen for gastroesophageal reflux disease based upon frequency of 12 common symptoms

#Adjusted for age, sex, race, known atherosclerotic risk factors (hypertension, diabetes, hyperlipidemia, and tobacco use)

†Adjusted for strong correlates of AF: ischemic heart disease, cardiomyopathy, atrial septal defect, status post coronary bypass surgery

AF= atrial fibrillation; aRR= adjusted relative risk; GERD= gastroesophageal reflux disorder; HR= hazard ratio; PAF= paroxysmal atrial fibrillation; PPI= proton pump inhibitor; RR= relative risk; USA= United States of America

Table 3. Relationship Between Atrial Fibrillation and Gastroesophageal-Like Symptoms

inhibitors (although the researchers did not have data medication use to test this hypothesis). Finally, the most recently published study assessed the relationship between atrial fibrillation and gastroesophageal reflux disease in 188 Japanese patients between 28-91 years of age [18]. Patients' gastroesophageal reflux disease status was classified using the F-scale, a questionnaire specifically designed to screen for gastroesophageal reflux disease. Almost half of

http://dx.doi.org/10.5772/56564

enrolled patients had a diagnosis of atrial fibrillation (n = 86), and while hypertension, dyslipidemia or coronary artery disease were not associated with the prevalence of symptomatic gastroesophageal reflux disease (defined as a total F-scale≥8 points) upon multivariate analysis, atrial fibrillation did show a significant correlation with gastroesophageal reflux disease ($p<0.001$). In addition, both the dyspeptic sub-score ($p=0.018$) and the total F-scale score ($p=0.019$) of atrial fibrillation patients were significantly greater than those in normal sinus rhythm.

Recognizing patients with both cardiovascular diseases and upper gastrointestinal conditions is an important step in their medical care. As demonstrated in available evidence, the links between the conditions are strong, and can impact therapeutic decisions.

3. Shared risk factors

The World Health Organization, World Heart Federation [1] and the American Heart Association [3] each agree on a set of risk factors for the development of cardiovascular diseases. These risk factors include smoking, being overweight or obese, living a sedentary lifestyle, and poor diet, as well as having pre-existing diagnoses of high cholesterol, hypertension and diabetes.

In addition to significantly contributing to the risk of developing cardiovascular disease, these same risk factors have also been found in epidemiologic studies to be associated with an increased risk of reporting upper gastrointestinal symptoms. These risk factors are highly prevalent both worldwide and in the United States [1,3].

Below we discuss the mechanism behind, and studies supporting, the association between these risk factors and increased rates of upper gastrointestinal symptoms.

3.1. Current smoking

Over a billion people worldwide are thought to be current smokers. It is estimated that nearly six million people die from tobacco-related deaths annually, and by 2030, this number is projected to surpass 8 million. Smoking is the underlying cause of about 10% of cardiovascular disease [1] and has been consistently found to be a strong and independent risk factor for myocardial infarction and sudden death [2]. Similar findings have been observed with cerebrovascular disease and smoking; with smokers having a 2 to 4 times increased risk of stroke compared with nonsmokers [2]. Consequently, it is not surprising that a large number of studies support the beneficial cardiovascular consequences of smoking cessation [1].

It is theorized that tobacco smoking/use induces upper gastrointestinal symptoms through its effects on the gastric mucosa [19]. The nicotine in tobacco likely causes mucosal injury by augmenting acid and pepsin release, causing duodenogastric reflux and producing free radicals; while at the same time decreasing prostaglandin and mucus production. Additionally, smoking may reduce lower esophageal sphincter pressure and thus accentuate gastroesophageal-like dyspeptic symptoms.

Risk Factor	Worldwide Prevalence Rate*	United States Prevalence Rate†
Current smoking	10%-31%	19.0%
Overweight (BMI>25 kg/m^2)	34%	34.6%
Obesity (BMI>30 kg/m^2)	9.8% (men)/13.8% (women)	34.6%
Insufficient physical activity (<150 minutes of moderate physical activity/week)	31.3%	21.0%
Poor diet patterns (<4 of 5 DASH-diet components)	N/A	79.0%
High cholesterol (Total cholesterol >240 mg/dL)	9.7%	13.8%
High blood pressure (≥140 SBP/≥90 DBP)	40%	33%
Diabetes (Fasting glucose ≥126 mg/dL)	10%	11.8%

*Rates per the World Heart Federation/World Health Organization [1]

†Rates per the American Heart Association [2]

BMI=body mass index; DASH=Dietary Approaches to Stop Hypertension; DBP=diastolic blood pressure; N/A=not available; SBP=systolic blood pressure

Table 4. Worldwide and United States-Specific Prevalence of Risk Factors for Cardiovascular Disease

While not consistently shown in every study [20-22], smoking's correlation with an increased upper gastrointestinal symptom prevalence (compared to abstainers) has been demonstrated to exist in a fair number of observational studies [8,20,23-25].

In an Australian study of 592 survey respondents of which 78 were dyspeptic, smoking was found to significantly increase this risk of reporting dyspeptic symptoms by more than 100% [19]. The Domestic/International Gastroenterology Surveillance Study also demonstrated smoking to be associated with a significantly greater prevalence of upper gastrointestinal symptoms (16% increase in relative risk) compared to those whom abstained from smoking; with the results of multivariate analysis suggesting smoking's largest negative effect was on heartburn and regurgitation (gastroesophageal-like) symptom prevalence [8].

Similar results were observed in two studies of United States veterans. In the first study, tobacco use was found to be associated with more symptoms of dyspepsia (odds ratio=1.31, 95% confidence interval, 1.03-1.66)[29]. In the second study, a 62% relative in-

http://dx.doi.org/10.5772/56564

Study, Year (N=)	Study Description	Key Finding
Nandurkar 1998 (N=592)	Healthy blood donors in Sydney, Australia completing the Bowel Symptoms Questionnaire; prevalence rate of upper gastrointestinal symptoms=13.2%	Smoking was an independent risk factor for dyspeptic symptoms (OR=2.1, 95%CI=1.3-3.6)
Stranghelli 1999 (N=5,581)	Respondents of the Domestic/International Gastroenterology Surveillance Study which surveyed urban, adult populations from 10 countries representing seven geographic areas (Canada, the USA, Switzerland, The Netherlands, Italy, Japan and the Nordic countries) using a study-specific symptom checklist; prevalence rate of upper gastrointestinal symptoms=28%	Prevalence rate of upper gastrointestinal symptoms were 30.8% for smokers and 26.5% for non-smokers, p=0.0003; Upon multivariate regression analysis, p<0.05 only for the relationship between smoking and gastroesophageal-like symptoms (p=0.03) and not ulcer- or dysmotility-like symptoms
Dominitz 1999 (N=1,582)	Respondents completing surveys (modified Bowel Disease Questionnaire) at one of 4 Durham, NC, USA Veterans Administration clinics; prevalence rate of upper gastrointestinal symptoms=30% (general medicine) to 53% (gastroenterology) depending on site of recruitment	Tobacco use was significantly associated with dyspeptic symptoms (OR=1.31, 95%CI=1.03-1.66)
Locke 1999 (N=1,524)	Cross-sectional survey study of Olmstead County, Minnesota residents completing the gastroesophageal reflux questionnaire; prevalence rate of frequent upper gastrointestinal symptoms=20%	Multivariate adjusted RR=1.3, 95%CI=0.8-2.1 for current vs. never smokers and OR=1.6, 95% confidence interval, 1.1-2.3 for past vs. never smoker
Shaib 2004 (N=465)	Employees of the Houston Veterans Affairs Medical Center, Texas, USA, completing the Gastro Esophageal Reflux Questionnaire; prevalence rate of upper gastrointestinal symptoms=31.4%	41.4% of dyspeptics (including those with gastroesophageal-like symptoms) were smokers vs. 25.6% non-dyspeptics; when gastroesophageal-like symptoms were excluded, no significant relationship between dyspeptic symptoms and smoking was seen (p=0.2)

CI=confidence interval; OR=odds ratio; RR=relative risk

Table 5. Summary of Studies Suggesting an Association Between Smoking and Upper Gastrointestinal Symptoms

crease in dyspepsia symptom reporting in smokers (41.4%) compared to non-smokers (25.6%) was observed. Again, as in the Domestic/International Gastroenterology Surveillance Study [8], subanalysis of the latter study suggested tobacco smoking may have a more profound effect on heartburn and regurgitation symptoms, as evidenced by the fact that the relationship between smoking and upper gastrointestinal symptom prevalence was no longer statistically significant when patients suffering gastroesophageal-like symptoms (~50% of the study population) were excluded from the analysis (p=0.2). This finding is further supported by a survey study conducted in Olmstead County, Minnesota where residents demonstrating current or past smoking increased respondents' risk of gastroesophageal symptoms by 30-60% [25].

3.2. Overweight or obesity

Overweight (body mass index ≥25 kg/m^2) or obesity (body mass index ≥30 kg/m^2) are highly prevalent disorders worldwide and are particular problems in the United States [1,3]. Obesity is strongly related to major cardiovascular risk factors such as elevated blood pressure, glucose intolerance, type 2 diabetes and dyslipidemia. Prospective studies have shown a significant relationship between overweight or obesity and an increased rate of cardiovascular events. In a collaborative meta-analysis of 58 cohorts (221,934 people from 17 countries, 14,297 incident cardiovascular disease outcomes, 1.87 million person-years at risk), patients' risk of coronary heart disease, ischemic stroke and cardiovascular disease were found to increase by 29%, 20% and 23%, respectively, for every 4.56 kg/m^2 increase in body mass index after adjustment for age, gender, and smoking status [26].

The mechanism behind the association between overweight/obesity and increased upper gastrointestinal symptoms is likely multifactorial [22]. First, the poor diet (ie, increased intake of fatty foods) [22] and lack of exercise that leads the overweight/obese state also promotes increased upper gastrointestinal symptoms (see further discussion below). Next, it is possible that abdominal obesity may lead to gastric compression by the surrounding adipose tissue. This causes increased intragastric pressure and relaxation of the lower esophageal sphincter, and ultimately heartburn and regurgitation. Obesity may also lead to the development of hiatal hernia promoting regurgitation symptoms. Lastly, humoral mechanisms related to obesity including increased levels of insulin, leptin, growth factors or hormones may contribute to gastrointestinal symptoms as well [22,27].

Results of the Domestic/International Gastroenterology Surveillance Study [3] suggested that the prevalence of upper gastrointestinal symptom reporting was higher in those with larger body mass indices. However, consistent with the proposed mechanisms listed above, it appeared the majority of the increased symptom burden related to increased body mass was gastroesophageal-like in nature.

In a meta-analysis of 9 studies examining the association between body mass index and gastroesophogeal-like symptoms, six (67%) found a statistically significant association. Furthermore, data from 8 of the 9 studies demonstrated a "dose-response relationship" between body mass index and gastroesophageal symptoms, with an increase in the pooled adjusted odds ratios for symptoms of 1.43 (95% confidence interval, 1.158 to 1.774) for body mass index of 25 kg/m^2 to 30 kg/m^2 and 1.94 (95% confidence interval, 1.468 to 2.566) for body mass index ≥ 30 kg/m^2 [28].

http://dx.doi.org/10.5772/56564

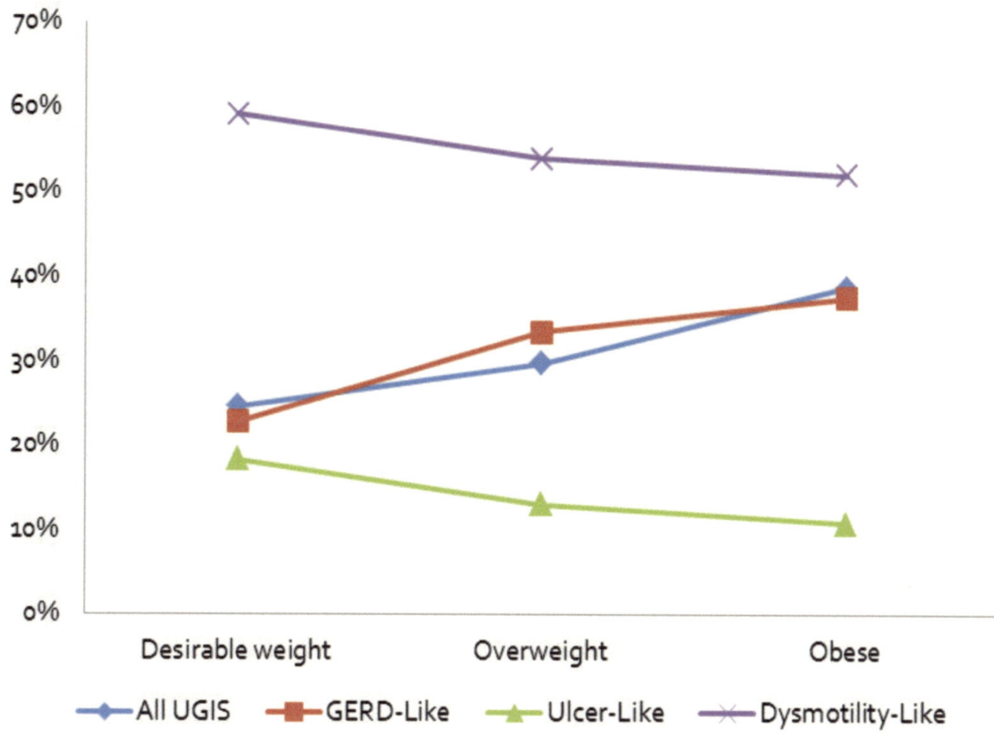

UGIS=upper gastrointestinal symptoms

Figure 2. Prevalence of Upper Gastrointestinal Symptoms (By Subtype) By Body Mass Index in the Domestic/International Gastroenterology Surveillance Study [3] Gastroesophogeal-like symptoms are the only symptom subtype trending upwards with increasing body mass index

3.3. Insufficient physical activity

Current guidance [1,29] recommends all adults should do at least 150 minutes a week of moderate-intensity aerobic physical activity, 75 minutes a week of vigorous-intensity aerobic physical activity, or some equivalent combination of both in order to reduce their risk of heart disease and diabetes. In fact, maintaining this level of moderate- or vigorous-intensity physical activity each week has been associated with as much as a 30% decrease in ischemic heart disease risk and a similar reduction (27%) in the risk of developing diabetes. Unfortunately, nearly a third of people worldwide and a fifth of Americans do not meet this goal [1,3]. While the mechanism behind how insufficient physical activity/sedentary lifestyle is associated with upper gastrointestinal symptoms is unclear, it may be that there is a higher rate of overweight/obesity in those who do not engage in enough physical activity, or the failure of inactive people to obtain the mental (reduced stress, reduced depressive symptoms and increased cognitive function) and bodily health benefits borne from physical activity [29].

Limited data evaluating the impact of physical activity on the prevalence of upper gastrointestinal symptoms have been published in the medical literature. In an internet survey of over

2,500 respondents complaining of functional dyspepsia (or other gastrointestinal symptoms), only 6% of respondents reported exercising daily, 29% reported exercising at least once a week, and a majority (54%) claimed almost never or never exercising [30]. This was significantly less physical activity compared to a simultaneously surveyed control population (n=1,000) ($p<0.01$), suggesting that a sedentary lifestyle may be associated with an increased prevalence of upper gastrointestinal symptoms.

3.4. Poor diet patterns

Improper or poor diet has been shown to be an important risk factor for cardiovascular disease. From a strict cardiovascular viewpoint an ideal diet consists the consumption of ≥4.5 cups per day of fruits and vegetables, ≥2 servings a week of fish, and ≥3 servings per day of whole grains and no more than 36 ounces per week of sugar-sweetened beverages and 1500 mg per day of sodium [31]. In addition, other poor diet choices such as high dietary intake of saturated fat, trans-fat and cholesterol have also been tied to poor cardiovascular outcomes [1].

The failure to meet the above-mentioned dietary and lifestyle goals not only hinders a person's ability to achieve a healthy body weight, desirable cholesterol profile, and blood pressure, but has also been linked to increased rates of upper gastrointestinal complaints. In a retrospective database analysis [9] of employed Americans with functional dyspepsia determined by having an ICD-9 code of 536.8x (n=1,669) and matched controls (n=83,450), those found to have a nutritional deficiency (defined by the Agency of Healthcare Research and Quality's Clinical Classifications Software grouping of relevant ICD-9 codes) were 3.8-times as likely to complain of dyspeptic symptoms ($p<0.05$). Moreover, in the previously mentioned survey study of >2,500 respondents complaining of dyspeptic or irritable bowel symptoms and 1,000 controls [30], the irregular eating of meals was found to be associated with increased gastrointestinal complaints ($p<0.05$).

A handful of observational studies have also more specifically evaluated the individual contributions of various components of poor diet on upper gastrointestinal symptom prevalence. An insufficient intake of vegetables has been found to be statistically significantly associated with increased gastrointestinal complaints ($p<0.05$) [30]. Moreover, in a sample of 1,000 employees of the United States Veteran's Administration system, a strong trend ($p=0.09$) towards an increased prevalence of heartburn and regurgitation symptoms (adjusted odds ratio=1.71, 95% confidence interval, 0.92-3.17) in those with high intake of saturated fat (measured using the 100-item Block Food Frequency Questionnaire) was also observed [22].

3.5. High cholesterol and high blood pressure

Ten percent of the world's adult population (and nearly 14% of the United States population) have high cholesterol (total cholesterol ≥240 mg/dL) and more than one-third of all people have high blood pressure (systolic and diastolic blood pressure ≥140 and 90 mm Hg, respectively), including 77.9 million American adults. Approximately one third of the global burden of ischemic heart disease can be attributed to high cholesterol, and each 20/10 mmHg increase in blood pressure, starting at 115/75 mmHg, has been shown to double a patients' risk of a cardiovascular event. The treatment of both high cholesterol and high blood pressure often necessitates polypharmacy [32,33], and many of the drugs used to treat these conditions may cause upper gastrointestinal symptoms (see further discussion below).

There are conflicting data regarding the association between high cholesterol, high blood pressure and upper gastrointestinal symptoms. In one recent retrospective database analysis of 4-years' worth of data on 300,000 employees of companies in the United States-based, patients with ICD-9 codes for functional dyspepsia symptoms (n=1,669) were found to have a higher rate of both high cholesterol (prevalence rates of 21.2% versus 12.1%, $p<0.05$) and essential hypertension (17.8% versus 12.4%, $p<0.05$) compared to matched controls without upper gastrointestinal symptom coding (n=83,450) [9]. However, in a far older study examining nearly 5,000 adults in the Rand Health Experiment, no statistically significant association was observed between either hypercholesterolemia or hypertension and patient reporting of "episodes or attacks of stomach pain or stomachache" in the prior 3-months [11].

3.6. Diabetes

In 2008, the global prevalence of diabetes (fasting plasma glucose ≥ 126 mg/dL) was estimated to be 10%, resulting in approximately 1.3 million deaths. A diagnosis of diabetes increases patients' risk of cardiovascular disease by 2- to 3-fold, and consequently, cardiovascular disease accounts for approximately 60% of all diabetes-related deaths [1].

Diabetes may increase peoples' risk of having upper gastrointestinal complaints for a number of reasons. First, many medications used to treat diabetes and hopefully reduce patient's risk of both cardiovascular and microvascular (retinopathy, neuropathy, nephropathy) complications can cause upper gastrointestinal symptoms including biguanides, sulfonylureas and alpha-glucosidase inhibitors [34]. Next, abnormal glucose regulation tends to occur in conjunction with other cardiovascular risk factors such as obesity, elevated blood pressure, low high-density lipoprotein cholesterol and a high triglyceride levels [1], as well as psychiatric disorders [35]; all known to be risk factors for upper gastrointestinal symptoms. Finally, the neuropathy associated with diabetes and resulting gastroparesis may cause diabetics to suffer from more upper gastrointestinal problems [35]. A recent prospective cohort study of 782 individuals found that *Helicobacter pylori* infection (a common cause of upper gastrointestinal symptoms) was associated with a 2.69-fold increased hazard of developing type II diabetes (95% confidence interval=1.10-6.60) [36], suggesting the relationship between diabetes and upper gastrointestinal symptoms may be bidirectional.

Some studies support the association between diabetes and upper gastrointestinal symptoms. The Domestic/International Gastroenterology Surveillance Study demonstrated those suffering from a metabolic or endocrine disorder (which would presumably include in large part, diabetes) were 2.6- to 4.4-fold more likely to report upper gastrointestinal symptoms in the prior three months ($p<0.006$)[8]. A study of Swedish type II diabetics (n=61) and non-diabetics (n=106) asked to complete a gastrointestinal symptom checklist found type II diabetes were more likely to report abdominal pain more often than once a month (28.3% versus 14.3%, $p<0.01$) and heartburn (31.77% versus 14.0%, $p<0.05$) [37]. Interestingly, it appears that the prevalence of upper gastrointestinal symptoms in diabetics may be linked to the extent/

severity of their disease, with a large (n=1,101) cross-sectional survey study demonstrating higher adjusted odds of frequent abdominal pain (odds ratio=1.62, 95% confidence interval, 1.02-2.58), dysmotility-like dyspepsia (odds ratio=2.01, 95% confidence interval, 1.30-3.11), ulcer-like dyspepsia (odds ratio=1.49, 95% confidence interval, 0.90-2.45) and gastroesophageal reflux symptoms (odds ratio=2.28, 95% confidence interval, 1.54-3.38) in patients experiencing a diabetes-related complication compared to those whom did not, and higher adjusted odds of dysmotility-like dyspepsia (odds ratio=1.32, 95% confidence interval, 1.08-1.60), ulcer-like dyspepsia (odds ratio=1.36, 95% confidence interval, 1.06-1.75) in those with poorer hemoglobin A1c control [38].

Appropriate management of the overlapping risk factors can result in additional benefit to the patients. Of the many care management decisions to be made between the health care providers and the patients, an understanding of the risk factor pattern can help with the prioritization. These overlapping risk factors may deserve a higher priority, as they will improve both the cardiovascular and upper gastrointestinal conditions at the same time.

4. Overlapping symptomatology and surveillance

As many as 40% of people will complain of chest pain (along with associated symptoms of nausea, palpitations and shortness of breath) at least once in their lifetime [39,48]; however, symptoms reported by patients are typically unreliable for differentiating between chest pain of a cardiac or gastrointestinal (ie, dyspepsia, gastroesophageal reflux, peptic ulcer disease, pancreatitis, cholecystitis) origin [39,49]. Hence, the birth of famous adages such as, "*when a young man complains of pain in his heart, it is usually his stomach; when an old man complains of pain in his stomach, it is usually his heart*" [39]. Upper gastrointestinal symptoms, particularly gastroesophageal- or dysmotility-like dyspeptic symptoms, are a frequent cause of non-cardiac chest pain (ie, recurrent episodes of substernal chest pain in patients lacking a cardiac diagnosis after a comprehensive evaluation) [39]. This likely explains why as many as 55% of chest pain suffers presenting to the emergency room for the first time are not ultimately diagnosed with cardiovascular disease [50], and 30% of patients undergoing coronary angiography each year show no signs of coronary heart disease [51]. However, despite the lack of a cardiac diagnosis, up to 80% of non-cardiac chest pain sufferers continue to experience symptoms over time, and 25%-45% continue to take antianginal medications [52]. Thus, because of the critical and continual need to differentiate between cardiovascular disease and upper gastrointestinal symptoms in patients with chest pain, it would seem reasonable to assume the increased surveillance of one of these disorders would result in a higher rate of diagnosis of the other.

It has been suggested that in areas with a high prevalence of *H. pylori* infection, a "search and treat" strategy for ischemic heart disease patients with dyspepsia could significantly reduce the need for urgent postoperative endoscopy due to major gastrointestinal events [53]. However, endoscopy has been shown to induce cardiovascular complications, including myocardial ischemia [40,41,54]. Thus, this practice may serve as an additional explanation for the frequent diagnosis of cardiovascular disease in patients experiencing upper gastrointestinal symptoms. An early study [54] of 110,469 upper endoscopies performed by 82 gastroenterologists and 12 internists found a rate of 5 cardiopulmonary complications (not specifically defined) per 100,000 procedures performed. However, more recent studies in patients with stable coronary disease or those at risk for cardiovascular disease have observed much higher rates of cardiovascular complications following endoscopy. In a study of 71 patients with stable coronary heart disease undergoing endoscopy for evaluation for the safety of secondary prophylaxis with aspirin, 42% of patients experienced silent ischemia and one patient had a symptomatic event [40]. A second study utilizing data from 9 hospitals in the United States evaluated 602 charts for patients undergoing endoscopy and deemed to be at risk for cardiovascular disease. The researchers found an overall cardiovascular complication (either an arrhythmia, hypotension, chest pain or angina equivalent, or myocardial infarction requiring intervention and occurring within one calendar day after the endoscopy) rate of one for every 325 procedures (or 308 complications per 100,000), and a rate as high as one complication for every 94 procedures (1,063 complications per 100,000) at the worst performing hospital [41]; a complication rate 2- to 70-fold higher than previously reported in the medical literature.

The awareness of how the symptoms of cardiovascular diseases and upper gastrointestinal conditions overlap can improve the differential diagnosis, thus reducing the chance of inappropriate procedures and medications.

5. Adverse effect of cardiovascular drugs

Optimal treatment of patients with cardiovascular disease [32,33] often requires the use of multiple medications. Consequently, at least some of the burden of upper gastrointestinal symptoms experienced in patients suffering from cardiovascular disease may be a result of polypharmacy. In the aforementioned Domestic/International Gastroenterology Surveillance Study [8], the occurrence of upper gastrointestinal symptoms was significantly higher in respondents reporting the use of a prescribed medication for another health problem compared to those not prescribed a medication (10.6% versus 6.0%, 5.1% versus 3.5% and 19.1% versus 13.3% for gastroesophogeal-, ulcer- and dysmotility-like symptoms, respectively, multivariate $p<0.007$ for all). Likewise, the use of an over-the-counter medication was also associated with a higher rate of upper gastrointestinal symptoms in general and dysmotility-like symptoms (19.3% versus 13.2% and 33.9% versus 24.6%; $p<0.0001$ for both).

Numerous drugs indicated or commonly used to treat cardiovascular diseases including antiplatelets, antiarrhythmics, antihypertensives, antianginals, cholesterol-lowering medications, as well as drugs to manage heart failure, diabetes and chronic kidney disease have been linked to the development of upper gastrointestinal symptoms.

Unfortunately, drug-induced dyspepsia can be difficult to identify because of the high background reporting of upper gastrointestinal symptoms. To overcome this problem, two studies [42,43,45] were conducted in a Dutch prescription database of over 1.5 million prescriptions (92 million person-years of follow-up) to identify signals for drug-induced dyspepsia using prescription sequence symmetry analysis methods. The basic principle behind these types of analyses is that most patients complaining of drug-induced dyspeptic symptoms are empirically treated with anti-ulcer and/or anti-dysmotility agents; therefore, a drug's propensity for causing upper gastrointestinal symptoms might be reflected in the sequencing of anti-ulcer and/or anti-dysmotility agents relative to the other medication (eg, an excess of patients presenting with their first prescription for an anti-ulcer or dysmotility agent after compared to before the initiation of an index drug would suggest a possible dyspepsia-causing effect of the index drug). These studies identified a handful of (index) drugs to treat cardiovascular disease that were more often followed by (within 100-days), as compared to preceded by a histmaine-2-antagonist, proton pump inhibitor, bismuth preparation, sucralfate, cispiride or metoclopramide. Drugs used to treat heart failure were among the drugs with the largest relative risks for upper gastrointestinal symptoms.

Cardiovascular Drug(s)	Common Cardiovascular Indication(s)
Acetylsalicylic acid (and other NSAIDs)	Antiplatelet
Amiodarone	Antiarrhythmic
Amlodipine (and other calcium channel blockers)	Antihypertensive, antianginal
Atorvastatin (and other statins)	High cholesterol
Beta-blockers	Antihypertensive, antianginal, heart failure
Bile acid sequestrants (less often with colesevelam)	High cholesterol
Non-aspirin antiplatelet agents (ie, cilostazol, ticlopidine)	Antiplatelet
Fibric acid derivatives (gemfibrozil>fenofibrate)	High cholesterol
Fish oil preparations (ie, omega-3 fatty acids)	High cholesterol, dietary supplement
Digoxin	Atrial fibrillation, heart failure
Dronedarone	Antiarrhythmic (atrial fibrillation)
Loop diuretics	Heart failure, chronic kidney disease
Losartan	Antihypertensive, heart failure, diabetes, chronic kidney disease
Niacin and nicotinic acid derivatives	High cholesterol
Nitrates	Antianginal
Potassium supplements	Dietary supplement
Ramipril (and other ACE inhibitors)	Antihypertensive, heart failure, diabetes, chronic kidney disease

This list was derived from searches of references 41,42,44,54,55

ACE=angiotensin-converting enzyme; NSAID=non-steroidal anti-inflammatory

Table 6. Cardiovascular Drugs Commonly Associated With Upper Gastrointestinal Symptoms

While a plausible explanation or underlying mechanism by which the abovementioned cardiovascular drugs can cause upper gastrointestinal symptoms is not always apparent, these drugs likely induce symptoms through direct mucosal irritation or injury (ie, aspirin and other non-steroidal anti-inflammatory drugs, potassium supplementation), facilitation of gastric acid reflux (ie, calcium channel blockers, nitrates) or alteration of gastric motility (ie, drugs targeting the renin-angiotensin system causing bradykinin-mediated dysmotility) [45,55]. Still yet, other associations between cardiovascular drugs and upper gastrointestinal symptoms may be "false" signals, representing nothing more than a link between a specific disease state or other confounder and upper gastrointestinal symptoms. Such may be the case with cholesterol-lowering medications. Patients with hypercholesterolemia may prefer frequent consumption of high-fat meals a well-known independent predictors of higher gastroesophageal symptom prevalence rates. [22,42,43,45].

Similarly, while drugs commonly used to treat heart failure, including angiotensin-converting enzyme inhibitors, angiotensin receptor blockers, loop diuretics and digoxin, have also been demonstrated in prescription sequence symmetry analyses to be upper gastrointestinal symptom-inducing; it is likely the symptoms attributed to them are a manifestation of heart failure itself (which has previously been shown to increase the risk of ulcer-like symptoms by as much as 3.6-fold [11]) and not the individual medications [11,57]. Of note, this may not always be the case with digoxin, which has been associated with dyspeptic-like symptoms in patients experiencing elevated/toxic blood concentrations (>2.0 ng/mL) [58].

Each year about 400,000 tons of aspirin (acetylsalicylic acid) are produced worldwide, and >50 million Americans take between 10 and 20 billion tablets for cardiovascular disease prevention [59]. Aspirin becomes non-ionized in the acidic environment of the gastrointestinal tract allowing it to penetrate mucosal tissue and cause irritation. Consequently it is not surprising that numerous studies have demonstrated aspirin to increase patients' relative risk of upper gastrointestinal symptoms by more than 2-fold over non-users [19-21,24,44]. Because of aspirin's frequent use and its propensity to cause gastric mucosal injury, it is likely the biggest drug-induced dyspepsia offender and one of the strongest links between upper gastrointestinal symptoms and cardiovascular disease. While it is best to stop aspirin in light of gastrointestinal symptoms, there may be adverse cardiovascular consequences that need to be considered. A double-blind, placebo-controlled study evaluating low-dose aspirin users who experienced gastrointestinal bleeding compared continuation of aspirin with discontinuation [60]. Seventy-eight patients received aspirin 80 mg daily while 78 received placebo daily for 8 weeks. All patients received intravenous followed by oral proton pump inhibitor therapy (intravenous pantoprazole 80 mg bolus followed by 8 mg/hour for 72 hours then oral pantoprazole 40mg daily). Recurrent bleeding occurred in 10.3% of patients in the aspirin group vs. 5.4% of those in the placebo group (difference=4.9 points, 95% confidence interval=-3.6 to 13.4), p=not significant), but patients who received aspirin had lower all-cause mortality rates than patients who received placebo (1.3% vs. 12.9%, difference=11.6 points, 95% confidence interval=3.7 to 19.5). As such, if aspirin must be part of the regimen, like in settings where dual antiplatelet therapy is needed (cardiac stenting, post unstable angina and myocardial infarction), treating the adverse gastrointestinal effects may be a superior strategy.

Index Cardiovascular Drugs	N Incident Users in Background	UGIS Drug First/Last	ARR (95% CI)
H2A, PPI, Bismuth, Sucralfate			
Digoxin	6,883	118/151	1.25 (0.99, 1.61)
Nitrates	10,661	220/241	1.08 (0.90, 1.30)
CCBs	15,940	224/315	1.40 (1.18, 1.67)
ACE inhibitors	12,097	143/192	1.38 (1.12, 1.73)
Cispiride			
Digoxin	6,883	18/11	1.52 (0.78, 3.57)
ACE inhibitors	12,097	21/16	1.28 (0.71, 2.62)
Metoclopramide			
Potassium supplement	16,933	194/130	1.42 (1.15, 1.79)
Digoxin	6,883	103/35	2.87 (2.01, 4.35)
Nitrates	10,661	56/32	1.74 (1.16, 2.77)
Loop diuretics	19,383	234/149	1.50 (1.23, 1.85)
CCBs	15,940	71/55	1.29 (0.93, 1.88)
ACE inhibitors	12,097	53/24	2.27 (1.46, 3.85)

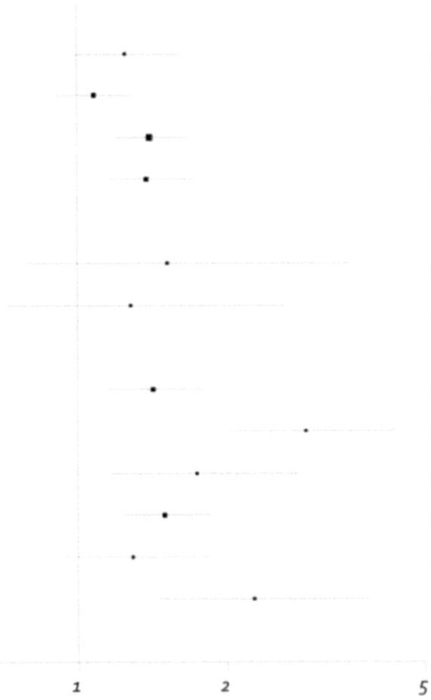

ACE=angiotensin-converting enzyme; ARR=adjusted rate ratios; CCBs=calcium channel blockers; CI=confidence intervals; H2A=histamine-2-antagonist; PPI=proton pump inhibitor; UGIS=upper gastrointestinal symptoms

Figure 3. Results of Cardiovascular Drug Sequence Symmetry Analyses Using Histmaine-2-Antagonists, Proton Pump Inhibitors, Bismuth Preparations or Sucralfate, Cispiride or Metoclopramide. The cardiovascular sequence symmetry analyses depicted above assumed the development of one or more upper gastrointestinal symptoms was followed by (within 100 days) the prescription of a drug to treat it (eg, a histmaine-2-antagonist, proton pump inhibitors, bismuth preparation or sucralfate, cispiride or metoclopramide). Results were reported as the adjusted rate ratio of individuals with AN upper gastrointestinal symptom-treating drug prescribed last versus individuals with the upper gastrointestinal symptom-treating drug prescribed first. Ratios above 1.0 indicate a possible upper gastrointestinal symptom-inducing effect of the index cardiovascular drug.

Of note, while studies suggest enteric-coated or buffered formulations of aspirin provide no significant protective effect against gastrointestinal complications [61], randomized trials of patients taking aspirin suggest concomitant proton pump inhibitor therapy can both prevent upper gastrointestinal symptoms ($p<0.05$) [62] and reduce their prevalence in patients already suffering dyspeptic symptoms [44,62].

Aspirin is not, however, the only antithrombotic agent that has been associated with upper gastrointestinal symptoms. In fact, both non-aspirin antiplatelet agents (including other non-steroidals, P2Y12 platelet inhibitors and phosphodiesterase inhibitors) and anticoagulants (particularly oral direct thrombin inhibitors) have been associated with clinically important

http://dx.doi.org/10.5772/56564

UGIS	PPI Group	Placebo Group
Epigastric pain	83.9%	66.7%*
Epigastric burning	72.7%	58.1%
Epigastric discomfort	68.3%	50.9%*
Heartburn	89.7%	66.7%*
Acid reflux	86.4%	56.5%*
Nausea	92.6%	78.6%
Bloating	77.9%	66.1%

*p≤0.05

PPI=proton pump inhibitor; UGIS=upper gastrointestinal symptoms

Table 7. Percentages of Patients Taking Aspirin (75-325 mg/day) and Suffering Upper Gastrointestinal Symptoms Reporting Resolution of Symptoms Following 26-Weeks of Proton Pump Inhibitor (Esomeprazole 20 mg/day) Therapy or Placebo [62]

rates of upper gastrointestinal symptoms [46,47,63]. In the largest systematic review to date (92 controlled trials), non-steroidals were found to increase the risk of dyspepsia versus placebo regardless of whether a strict (relative risk=1.36, 95% confidence interval=1.11-1.67) or liberal definition (relative risk= 1.19, 95% confidence interval=1.03-1.39) was used; with a placebo rate of 2.3% using the strict definition and 4.2% using the liberal definition [63].

In a systematic review of randomized controlled trials of adults with atrial fibrillation receiving pharmacologic stroke prevention, not only were upper gastrointestinal adverse effects found to be common place, but oral direct thrombin inhibitors were associated with highest incidences of (~11%) and drug discontinuation due to these symptoms (~2%) [46]. The Randomized Evaluation of Long-Term Anticoagulation Therapy (RE-LY) study found a statistically higher incidence of dyspepsia in patients receiving the oral direct thrombin inhibitor, dabigatran, compared to adjusted-dose warfarin (11.8% for dabigatran 110 mg, 11.3% for dabigatran 150 mg and 5.8% for warfarin, p<0.001 for the comparison of either dose of dabigatran versus warfarin)[47]. The dyspepsia-provoking nature of dabigatran has been attributed to its formulation which utilizes a tartaric acid core to lower the pH in the gastrointestinal tract and thus increase the absorption of the drug [47]. Luckily, there are Factor Xa inhibitors as therapeutic alternatives to direct thrombin inhibitors in those impacted by, or likely to be impacted by, upper gastrointestinal symptoms [56,64].

Beyond the ability of cardiovascular drugs to provoke upper gastrointestinal symptoms, the occurrence of these symptoms may adversely affect cardiovascular drug adherence, putting

Agent	Mechanism of Action	UGIS	Nausea
Antiplatelet agents			
ASA	Blockade of COX-1	++++ (>6%)	++++ (>6%)
Non-ASA NSAIDs	Blockade of COX-1	+++ (ibuprofen, naproxen: 2-3%); ++++ (indomethacin: >6%)	+++/++++ (drug dependent: 3-9%)
Cilostazol	PDE III blockade	++++ (~6%)	++++ (~7%)
Clopidogrel	P2Y12 inhibition	++ (<2%)	++ (<2%)
Prasugrel	P2Y12 inhibition	++ (<2%)	+++ (~5%)
Ticagrelor	P2Y12 inhibition	++ (~2%)	+++ (~4%)
Ticlopidine	P2Y12 inhibition	++++ (~7%)	++++ (~7%)
Anticoagulant agents			
Warfarin	Vitamin K antagonist	++++ (6%)	++ (1.5%)
Dabigatran	Direct thrombin inhibition	++++ (11%)	NA
Rivaroxaban	Factor Xa inhibition	++ (≤2%)	++ (2%)
Apixaban	Factor Xa inhibition	NA	+++ (3%)

++=minimal risk (≤2%); +++=moderate risk (3-5%); ++++=high risk (5-10%)

ASA=aspirin; COX=cyclooxygenase; NSAID=non-steroidal anti-inflammatory drug; NA=not available; PDE=phosphodiesterase; UGIS=upper gastrointestinal symptoms

Table 8. Cross-Comparison of Upper Gastrointestinal Symptoms Precipitated by Antithrombotics [46,47,56,65]

patients at risk for adverse cardiovascular outcomes. Studies have demonstrated that gastrointestinal side effects decrease medication adherence [66], and this likely plays an important role in the poor adherence often seen across the spectrum cardiovascular medications [67].

6. Cardiovascular disease associated with upper gastrointestinal symptom drug use

In addition to cardiovascular drugs provoking upper gastrointestinal symptoms, a number of medications used to treat upper gastrointestinal symptoms have impacted cardiovascular drug function or have been associated with poor cardiovascular outcomes through both indirect and direct mechanisms.

6.1. Drug interactions impeding cardiovascular drug function

Proton pump inhibitors are frequently used to treat various gastrointestinal symptoms/ conditions including *H. pylori* infection. American College of Gastroenterology guidelines recommended strategies for the eradication of *H. pylori* infection include treatment with at least three drugs, and yield eradication rates of up to 90%. While the best *H. pylori* treatment regimen may vary depending on patient characteristics, guidelines recommended four different drug regimens including a proton pump inhibitor, clarithromycin, and amoxicillin, or metronidazole (clarithromycin-based triple therapy) for 14 days, a proton pump inhibitor or histamine-2-antagonist, bismuth, metronidazole, and tetracycline (bismuth quadruple therapy) for 10–14 days, or sequential therapy consisting of a proton pump inhibitor and amoxicillin for 5 days followed by a proton pump inhibitor, clarithromycin, and tinidazole for an additional 5 days (as an alternative to clarithromycin-based triple or bismuth quadruple therapy) [68].

Proton pump inhibitors competitively inhibit the cytochrome P450 2C19 isoenzyme (CYP2C19). Based on in vitro and in vivo data, omeprazole and esomeprazole are the most potent CYP2C19 inhibitors [69]. In vivo, omeprazole and esomeprazole induced 4 and 10 fold functional inhibition of CYP2C19 versus less than 1.5 fold inhibition with lansoprazole and pantoprazole [70]. Rabeprazole has in vitro data showing less inhibition of CYP2C19 than omeprazole and lansoprazole but no in vivo data is available [69].

Clopidogrel is a CYP2C19 substrate and needs to be activated by this isoenzyme. When given concurrently with proton pump inhibitors, there is a reduction in the produced active form of clopidogrel and greater platelet reactivity (less platelet inhibition) [71,72].

Whether this platelet reactivity effect impacts clinical events has been controversial. A 2009 population-based study among Ontario residents aged 66 years or older used prescription records to ascertain proton pump inhibitor use during clopidogrel therapy. The analysis suggested that proton pump inhibitor use may be associated with an increased risk of cardiovascular events [odds ratio for recurrent myocardial infarction within 90 days following hospital discharge, 1.27 (1.03 to 1.57)], however, no effect on the risk of death was observed [odds ratio of death within 90 days following hospital discharge 0.82 (0.57 to 1.18)] [73]. The 16,718 patient Clopidogrel Medco Outcomes Study was a cohort evaluation from an integrated medical and pharmacy claims database. Patients had a clopidogrel prescription filled within one month of a coronary stenting procedure (where dual aspirin and clopidogrel therapy is frequently employed). Patients who concomitantly received a proton pump inhibitor were in the active group while those without were in the control group in this observational non-randomized study. Those receiving a proton pump inhibitor had more cardiovascular events (myocardial infarction, unstable angina, repeat coronary procedure) than those without (25% vs. 18%, $p<0.0001$). Without randomization, however, it cannot be ascertained where it was the underlying patient population with gastrointestinal symptoms that had a higher risk or if the use of the proton pump inhibitor yielded the difference. When patients on each proton pump inhibitor were analyzed separately, there were no differences in the percent of patients with a cardiac event: omeprazole 25%, esomeprazole 25%, lansoprazole 24%, and pantoprazole 29%. Given the marked differences in CYP2C19 inhibition between omeprazole and esomeprazole versus lansoprazole and pantoprazole, qualitative differences between the groups would have been expected [74]. Two other smaller analyses also supported the greater risk of cardiac events with patients receiving concurrent proton pump inhibitors but again, whether the additional risk is due to the underlying differences in the populations versus the use of the drug cannot be determined [75,76].

In the 13,608 patient TRITON-TIMI 38 Trial, a third of patients were on a concomitant proton pump inhibitor (41% pantoprazole, 37% omeprazole, 14% esomeprazole, 10% lansoprazole, 1% rabeprazole). In a nested cohort analysis from this trial, there was no difference between the proton pump inhibitor group and the control group for the composite endpoint of cardiovascular death, nonfatal myocardial infarction, or nonfatal stroke [77].

Given the profound effect of confounders, especially co-linear confounders, on the results of observational trials, these trials cannot prove causality, regardless of their results. Randomized and placebo controlled clinical trials eliminate many of these confounders and have much stronger internal validity. The only major randomized evaluation of the impact of proton pump inhibitors on cardiovascular events was the Clopidogrel and the Optimization of Gastrointestinal Events (COGENT) trial. Overall, 3761 patients starting dual antiplatelet therapy with aspirin and clopidogrel were randomized to receive omeprazole or placebo. No difference was found in the primary composite cardiovascular endpoint ($p=0.98$) but the rate of overt upper gastrointestinal bleeding was reduced with omeprazole therapy versus placebo [hazard ratio 0.13 (0.03 to 0.56)] [78]. The use of omeprazole which is the most potent CYP2C19 inhibitor was the best proton pump inhibitor choice to evaluate the balance of benefits to harms in this population [56, 69].

The COGENT trial and TRITON-TIMI 38 analysis results led the American College of Cardiology, American College of Gastroenterology, and American Heart Association to issue guidelines calling for the use of proton pump inhibitors when indicated for patients receiving antiplatelet therapy for cardiovascular disease [79]. However, the package insert recommends avoiding the use moderate to strong CYP2C19 inhibitors and to use alternative acid suppressing agents such as H2 antagonists or less potent CYP2C19 inhibiting proton pump inhibitors where possible [56].

Aside from proton pump inhibitors, the histamine-2 antagonist cimetidine is ubiquitous moderate CYP 1A2, 2C19, 2D6, and 3A4 inhibitor [56]. It raises the concentrations of all these cardiovascular medications increasing the chances for cardiovascular adverse effects. As such additional monitoring is suggested when added to amiodarone, beta-blockers (carvedilol, nebivolol), calcium channel clockers (verapamil, diltiazem, nifedipine), procainamide, propafenone, and ranolazine while selection of an alternative agent is specifically suggested when quinidine is being used. Other drugs in this class do not have the same potency of inhibition and are therapeutic alternatives [56].

6.2. QTc prolongation and Torsade de Pointes

Two classes of commonly used upper gastrointestinal drugs impact QTc prolongation and arrhythmogenesis. The QTc interval is a marker of ventricular depolarization and repolarization time and if the QTc interval reaches 500ms or is elevated by 60ms over baseline values, the risk of the polymorphic ventricular arrhythmia Torsade de Pointes is elevated [80]. Torsade de Pointes can be a life threatening arrhythmia and requires prompt detection and treatment.

http://dx.doi.org/10.5772/56564

Cisapride is a promotility agent that enhances acetylcholine release at the myenteric plexus [56]. In March of 2000, the Food and Drug Administration was notified that the manufacturer would stop widespread manufacture of the drug due to elevated risk of QTc interval prolongation and the formation of the polymorphic ventricular tachycardia Torsade de Pointes. There are 341 reports of heart rhythm abnormalities, likely Torsade de Pointes, and 80 deaths with cisapride. It is still being made and distributed to individuals for whom other options have failed but is contraindicated with QTc interval prolonging agents such as Vaughn Williams Class Ia (quinidine, procainamide) or Class III (amiodarone, dronedarone, sotalol, dofetilide) antiarrhythmic agents, macrolide antibiotics (erythromycin, clarithromycin, troleandomycin), nefazodone, HIV protease inhibitors, and -azole antifungals. It is also contraindicated with potent CYP3A4 inhibitors and prone individuals [56, 80]. While not classically considered a gastrointestinal drug, erythromycin stimulates motilin receptors and can be an adjunctive promotility agent in diabetic gastroparesis. Erythromycin blocks the rapid component of the delayed rectifier potassium channel and prolongs the QTc interval and arrhythmogenic risk as well [80].

The 5HT3 antagonists (dolasetron, granisetron, etc) prolong the QTc interval and when used intravenously or in patients with other QTc interval prolonging drugs, hypokalemia or hypomagnesemia, or congenital long QT syndrome; can induce the polymorphic ventricular arrhythmia known as Torsade de Pointes [80]. Correcting electrolyte abnormalities before starting a 5HT3 antagonist is important in preventing Torsade de Pointes but is also sometimes difficult given the emesis the drugs are being used to control [56].

6.3. Bradycardia and atrioventricular blockade

The 5HT3 antagonists (dolasetron, granisetron, ondansetron, etc) and the histamine 2 receptor antagonists (cimetidine, ranitidine) have been shown to rarely cause negative chronotropic (reduced sinoatrial nodal firing rate) and dromotropic (reduced rate of impulse passage through the atrioventricular node) effects when used in excessive doses or in intravenous forms [56, 80]. Patients who are prone to develop bradycardia or heart block, such as those with borderline low heart rates, elevated baseline PR intervals, or are receiving other negative chronotropic or dromotropic drugs (beta-blockers, nondihydropyridine calcium channel blockers, digoxin, Vaughn Williams Class Ic antiarrhythmic agents) are most at risk [56,80].

6.4. Hypertension

Metoclopramide is a complex dopaminergic agent with differing effects on blood pressure in different individuals. When used as a sole agent in normotensive, essential hypertensive, and type 2 diabetic subjects, there is no effect on systolic or diastolic blood pressure [81,82]. However, it can profoundly elevate blood pressure in patients with pheochromocytoma and in patients developing serotonin syndrome while taking metoclopramide with select serotonin reuptake inhibitors [83-86]. In addition, it has been shown to modestly attenuate the antihypertensive effects of bromocriptine and labetolol [87,88]. In this way, metoclopramide can induce hypertensive urgencies and emergencies in prone individuals and alternative agents should be utilized when appropriate.

The consequences of these drug-disease interactions can be dire, with significant impact on mortality and morbidities. As many of these interactions are unknown until a large population has been using the offending medications, health care providers must remain vigilant in identifying potential new problems.

7. Conclusions

There is growing evidence that patients with cardiovascular disease suffer a higher burden of upper gastrointestinal symptoms and even that certain upper gastrointestinal complaints can induce or promote cardiovascular disease. Knowledge of how these common conditions are connected can bring forth therapeutic advantages. For instance, among patients with upper gastrointestinal symptoms, their interactions with the health care system can increase the chance of earlier diagnosis of cardiovascular conditions. Conversely, among patients with cardiovascular conditions, health care providers' inquiry into gastrointestinal symptoms and side effects of medications may aid in appropriate choice of therapy to enhance effectiveness and patient adherence. Additional research is needed to clarify whether the cardiovascular patients' increased risk of upper gastrointestinal symptoms is a result of shared pathophysiology or risk factors, increased surveillance due to overlapping symptoms, or induced by the frequent need for polypharmacy among suffers of both these disease states.

Author details

Craig I. Coleman[1,2*], Brendan L. Limone[2], Jeff R. Schein[3], Winnie W. Nelson[3], Joyce C. LaMori[4], Jeffrey Kluger[5] and C. Michael White[1,2]

*Address all correspondence to: ccolema@harthosp.org

1 Department of Pharmacy Practice, University of Connecticut School of Pharmacy, Storrs, CT, USA

2 Evidence-Based Practice Center, Hartford Hospital, Hartford, CT, USA

3 Heath Economics and Outcomes Research; Janssen Scientific Affairs, Raritan, NJ, USA

4 Translational Science, Heath Economics and Outcomes Research; Janssen Scientific Affairs, Raritan, NJ, USA

5 Department of Cardiology, Hartford Hospital, Hartford, CT, USA

References

[1] World Health Organization. Global atlas on cardiovascular disease prevention and control. Available at: http://www.who.int/cardiovascular_diseases/en/ (Last accessed on December 29, 2012).

[2] Go AS, Mozaffarian D, Roger VL, Benjamin EJ, Berry JD, Borden WB, Bravata DM, Dai S, Ford ES, Fox CS, Franco S, Fullerton HJ, Gillespie C, Hailpern SM, Heit JA, Howard VJ, Huffman MD, Kissela BM, Kittner SJ, Lackland DT, Lichtman JH, Lisabeth LD, Magid D, Marcus GM, Marelli A, Matchar DB, McGuire DK, Mohler ER, Moy CS, Mussolino ME, Nichol G, Paynter NP, Schreiner PJ, Sorlie PD, Stein J, Turan TN, Virani SS, Wong ND, Woo D, Turner MB; on behalf of the American Heart Association Statistics Committee and Stroke Statistics Subcommittee. Heart disease and stroke statistics—2013 update: a report from the American Heart Association.*Circulation*.2013;127:e000-e000.

[3] Stanghellini V. Three-month prevalence rates of gastrointestinal symptoms and the influence of demographic factors: results from the Domestic/International Gastroenterology Surveillance Study (DIGEST). Scand J Gastroenterol Suppl. 1999;231:20-8.

[4] Haycox A, Einarson T, Eggleston A. The health economic impact of upper gastrointestinal symptoms in the general population: results from the Domestic/International Gastroenterology Surveillance Study (DIGEST). Scand J Gastroenterol Suppl. 1999;231:38-47.

[5] Drossman DA, Li Z, Andruzzi E, Temple RD, Talley NJ, Thompson WG, Whitehead WE, Janssens J, Funch-Jensen P, Corazziari E, et al. U.S. householder survey of functional gastrointestinal disorders. Prevalence, sociodemography, and health impact. Dig Dis Sci. 1993;38(9):1569-80.

[6] Enck P, Dubois D, Marquis P. Quality of life in patients with upper gastrointestinal symptoms: results from the Domestic/International Gastroenterology Surveillance Study (DIGEST). Scand J Gastroenterol Suppl. 1999;231:48-54.

[7] American Academy of Family Physicians. ICD-9 codes for Family Medicine 2011-2012: The FPM Short List. Available at: http://www.aafp.org/fpm/icd9/icd9-short.pdf (Last accessed on January 10, 2013).

[8] Stanghellini V. Relationship between upper gastrointestinal symptoms and lifestyle, psychosocial factors and comorbidity in the general population: results from the Domestic/International Gastroenterology Surveillance Study (DIGEST). Scand J Gastroenterol Suppl. 1999;231:29-37.

[9] Brook RA, Kleinman NL, Choung RS, Smeeding JE, Talley NJ. Excess comorbidity prevalence and cost associated with functional dyspepsia in an employed population. Dig Dis Sci. 2012;57(1):109-18.

[10] Wallander MA, Johansson S, Ruigómez A, García Rodríguez LA, Jones R. Dyspepsia in general practice: incidence, risk factors, comorbidity and mortality. Fam Pract. 2007;24(5):403-11.

[11] Lohr KN, Kamberg CJ, Keeler EB, Goldberg GA, Calabro TA, Brook RH. Chronic disease in a general adult population. Findings from the Rand Health Insurance Experiment. West J Med. 1986;145(4):537-45.

[12] LaMori JC, Mody SH, Gross HJ, DiBonaventura Md, Patel A, Schein J, Nelson WW. Dyspepsia and disease burden among patients with atrial fibrillation. Crit Pathw Cardiol. 2012;11(1):14-9.

[13] Laliberté F, Moore Y, Dea K, LaMori JC, Mody SH, Jones JL, Arledge MD, Damaraju CV, Duh MS, Schein JR, Lefebvre P. Risk of Gastrointestinal Conditions among Patients with Atrial Fibrillation. Pharmacoepidemiol Drug Saf. 2012;21(Suppl. 3): 264-265.

[14] Pasini GF, Melchioretti R, Mora A, Buizza MA, Almici CA, Davoli C, Pasini M, Alberti P. [Dyspeptic syndrome in heart diseases]. G Clin Med. 1989;70(2):101-4.

[15] Weigl M, Gschwantler M, Gatterer E, Finsterer J, Stöllberger C. Reflux esophagitis in the pathogenesis of paroxysmal atrial fibrillation: results of a pilot study. South Med J. 2003 Nov;96(11):1128-32.

[16] Kunz JS, Hemann B, Edwin Atwood J, Jackson J, Wu T, Hamm C. Is there a link between gastroesophageal reflux disease and atrial fibrillation? Clin Cardiol. 2009 Oct; 32(10):584-7.

[17] Bunch TJ, Packer DL, Jahangir A, Locke GR, Talley NJ, Gersh BJ, Roy RR, Hodge DO, Asirvatham SJ. Long-term risk of atrial fibrillation with symptomatic gastroesophageal reflux disease and esophagitis. Am J Cardiol. 2008 Nov 1;102(9):1207-11.

[18] Shimazu H, Nakaji G, Fukata M, Odashiro K, Maruyama T, Akashi K; Fukuoka F-Scale Trial Group. Relationship between atrial fibrillation and gastroesophageal reflux disease: a multicenter questionnaire survey. Cardiology. 2011;119(4):217-23.

[19] Nandurkar S, Talley NJ, Xia H, Mitchell H, Hazel S, Jones M. Dyspepsia in the community is linked to smoking and aspirin use but not to Helicobacter pylori infection. Arch Intern Med. 1998;158(13):1427-33.

[20] Talley NJ, Zinsmeister AR, Schleck CD, Melton LJ 3rd. Smoking, alcohol, and analgesics in dyspepsia and among dyspepsia subgroups: lack of an association in a community. Gut. 1994 May;35(5):619-24.

[21] Talley NJ, Weaver AL, Zinsmeister AR. Smoking, alcohol, and nonsteroidal anti-inflammatory drugs in outpatients with functional dyspepsia and among dyspepsia subgroups. Am J Gastroenterol. 1994;89(4):524-8.

[22] El-Serag HB, Graham DY, Satia JA, Rabeneck L. Obesity is an independent risk factor for GERD symptoms and erosive esophagitis. Am J Gastroenterol. 2005;100(6): 1243-1250.

[23] Dominitz JA, Provenzale D. Prevalence of dyspepsia, heartburn, and peptic ulcer disease in veterans. Am Gastroenterol. 1999;94(8):2086-2093.

[24] Shaib Y, El-Serag HB. The prevalence and risk factors of functional dyspepsia in a multiethnic population in the United States. Am J Gastroenterol. 2004;99(11): 2210-2216.

[25] Locke GR 3rd, Talley NJ, Fett SL, Zinsmeister AR, Melton LJ 3rd. Risk factors associated with symptoms of gastroesophageal reflux. Am J Med. 1999;106(6):642-9.

[26] Emerging Risk Factors Collaboration, Wormser D, Kaptoge S, Di Angelantonio E, Wood AM, Pennells L, Thompson A, Sarwar N, Kizer JR, Lawlor DA, Nordestgaard BG, Ridker P, Salomaa V, Stevens J, Woodward M, Sattar N, Collins R, Thompson SG, Whitlock G, Danesh J. Separate and combined associations of body-mass index and abdominal adiposity with cardiovascular disease: collaborative analysis of 58 prospective studies. Lancet. 2011;377(9771):1085-95.

[27] Infantino M. The prevalence and pattern of gastroesophageal refluxsymptoms in perimenopausal and menopausal women. J Am Acad Nurse Pract. 2008;20(5):266-272.

[28] Hampel H, Abraham NS, El-Serag HB. Meta-analysis: obesity and the risk for gastroesophageal reflux disease and its complications. Ann Intern Med. 2005;143(3): 199-211.

[29] United States Department of Health and Human Services. 2008 Physical Activity Guidelines for Americans. Available at: http://www.health.gov/paguidelines/guidelines/default.aspx (Last accessed on January 10, 2013).

[30] Miwa H. Life style in persons with functional gastrointestinal disorders--large-scale internet survey of lifestyle in Japan. Neurogastroenterol Motil. 2012;24(5):464-71, e217.

[31] United States Department of Agriculture and the United States Department of health and Human Services. Dietary Guidelines for Americans, 2010. Available at: http://www.dietaryguidelines.gov (Last accessed on January 10, 2013).

[32] Vandvik PO, Lincoff AM, Gore JM, Gutterman DD, Sonnenberg FA, Alonso-Coello P, Akl EA, Lansberg MG, Guyatt GH, Spencer FA; American College of Chest Physicians. Primary and secondary prevention of cardiovascular disease: Antithrombotic Therapy and Prevention of Thrombosis, 9th ed: American College of Chest Physicians Evidence-Based Clinical Practice Guidelines. Chest. 2012 Feb;141(2 Suppl):e637S-68S

[33] Smith SC Jr, Allen J, Blair SN, Bonow RO, Brass LM, Fonarow GC, Grundy SM, Hiratzka L, Jones D, Krumholz HM, Mosca L, Pasternak RC, Pearson T, Pfeffer MA,

Taubert KA; AHA/ACC; National Heart, Lung, and Blood Institute. AHA/ACC guidelines for secondary prevention for patients with coronary and other atherosclerotic vascular disease: 2006 update: endorsed by the National Heart, Lung, and Blood Institute. Circulation. 2006 May 16;113(19):2363-72.

[34] Inzucchi SE, Bergenstal RM, Buse JB, Diamant M, Ferrannini E, Nauck M, Peters AL, Tsapas A, Wender R, Matthews DR; American Diabetes Association (ADA); European Association for the Study of Diabetes (EASD). Management of hyperglycemia in type 2 diabetes: a patient-centered approach: position statement of the American Diabetes Association (ADA) and the European Association for the Study of Diabetes (EASD). Diabetes Care. 2012;35(6):1364-79.

[35] Koch CA, Uwaifo GI. Are gastrointestinal symptoms related to diabetes mellitus and glycemic control? Eur J Gastroenterol Hepatol. 2008;20(9):822-5.

[36] Jeon CY, Haan MN, Cheng C, Clayton ER, Mayeda ER, Miller JW, Aiello AE. Helicobacter pylori infection is associated with an increased rate of diabetes. Diabetes Care. 2012;35(3):520-5. doi: 10.2337/dc11-1043.

[37] Spångéus A, El-Salhy M, Suhr O, Eriksson J, Lithner F. Prevalence of gastrointestinal symptoms in young and middle-aged diabetic patients. Scand J Gastroenterol. 1999;34(12):1196-202.

[38] Bytzer P, Talley NJ, Hammer J, Young LJ, Jones MP, Horowitz M. gastrointestinal symptoms in diabetes mellitus are associated with both poor glycemic control and diabetic complications. Am J Gastroenterol. 2002;97(3):604-11.

[39] Simpson FG, Kay J, Aber CP. Chest pain--indigestion or impending heart attack? Postgrad Med J. 1984;60(703):338-40.

[40] Schenck J, Müller CH, Lübbers H, Mahlke R, Lehnick D, Lankisch PG. Does gastroscopy induce myocardial ischemia in patients with coronary heart disease? Endoscopy. 2000;32(5):373-6.

[41] Gangi S, Saidi F, Patel K, Johnstone B, Jaeger J, Shine D. Cardiovascular complications after gastrointestinal endoscopy: occurrence and risks in a large hospital system. Gastrointest Endosc. 2004;60(5):679-85.

[42] Hallas J, Bytzer P. Screening for drug related dyspepsia: an analysis of prescription symmetry. Eur J Gastroenterol Hepatol. 1998;10(1):27-32.

[43] Bytzer P, Hallas J. Drug-induced symptoms of functional dyspepsia and nausea. A symmetry analysis of one million prescriptions. Aliment Pharmacol Ther. 2000;14(11):1479-84.

[44] Laheij RJ, Jansen JB, Verbeek AL, Verheugt FW. Helicobacter pylori infection as a risk factor for gastrointestinal symptoms in patients using aspirin to prevent ischaemic heart disease. Aliment Pharmacol Ther. 2001;15(7):1055-9.

[45] Bytzer P. Dyspepsia as an adverse effect of drugs. Best Pract Res Clin Gastroenterol. 2010;24(2):109-20.

[46] Sobieraj DM, White CM, Alikhanov S, Winkler S, Mediouni M, Kluger J, Coleman CI. The impact of antiplatelet and anticoagulant therapies on gastrointestinal symptoms in patients with atrial fibrillation: a systematic review. Ann Pharmacother. 2012;46(9): 1220-31.

[47] Connolly SJ, Ezekowitz MD, Yusuf S, Eikelboom J, Oldgren J, Parekh A, Pogue J, Reilly PA, Themeles E, Varrone J, Wang S, Alings M, Xavier D, Zhu J, Diaz R, Lewis BS, Darius H, Diener HC, Joyner CD, Wallentin L; RE-LY Steering Committee and Investigators. Dabigatran versus warfarin in patients with atrial fibrillation. N Engl J Med. 2009;361(12):1139-51.

[48] Eslick GD, Jones MP, Talley NJ. Non-cardiac chest pain: prevalence, risk factors, impact and consulting--a population-based study. Aliment Pharmacol Ther. 2003;17(9): 1115-24.

[49] Kachintorn U. How do we define non-cardiac chest pain? J Gastroenterol Hepatol. 2005;20 Suppl:S2-5.

[50] Pope JH, Aufderheide TP, Ruthazer R, Woolard RH, Feldman JA, Beshansky JR, Griffith JL, Selker HP. Missed diagnoses of acute cardiac ischemia in the emergency department. N Engl J Med. 2000;342(16):1163-70.

[51] Katz PO, Castell DO. Approach to the patient with unexplained chest pain. Am J Gastroenterol. 2000;95(8 Suppl):S4-8.

[52] Tew R, Guthrie EA, Creed FH, Cotter L, Kisely S, Tomenson B. A long-term follow-up study of patients with ischaemic heart disease versus patients with nonspecific chest pain. J Psychosom Res. 1995;39(8):977-85.

[53] Banić M, Sutlić Z, Biocina B, Kujundzić M, Fabijanić D, Ljubicić N, Plesko S, Buljevac M, Kardum D, Cabrijan Z, Grgurević I, Urek M, Tadić M, Hulak V, Petrovecki M, Bedenikovic V, Starcević B, Rotkvić I. Peptic ulcer disease in dyspeptic patients with ischemic heart disease: search and treat? Z Gastroenterol. 2005;43(6):581-6.

[54] Sieg A, Hachmoeller-Eisenbach U, Eisenbach T. Prospective evaluation of complications in outpatient gastrointestinal endoscopy: a survey among German gastroenterologists. Gastrointest Endosc. 2001;53(6):620-7.

[55] Meyler's Side Effects of Drugs: The International Encyclopedia of Adverse Reactions and Interactions (Fifteenth Edition)

[56] Lexi-Drugs® with American Hospital Formulary Service Drug Information® Essentials™. Wolters Kluwer Health, 2012.

[57] Neil GA, Weinstock JV. Gastrointestinal manifestations of systemic diseases. In: Textbook of Gastroenterology. 2nd ed. Yamada et al. (editors). Philadelphia: JB Lippincott Company; 1995. p. 2420.

[58] Bauman JL, DiDomenico RJ, Galanter WL. Mechanisms, manifestations, and management of digoxin toxicity in the modern era. Am J Cardiovasc Drugs. 2006;6(2):77-86

[59] Fuster V, Sweeny JM. Aspirin: a historical and contemporary therapeutic overview. Circulation. 2011;123(7):768-78.

[60] Sung JJ, Lau JY, Ching JY, Wu JC, Lee YT, Chiu PW, et al. Continuation of low-dose aspirin therapy in peptic ulcer bleeding: a randomized trial. Ann Intern Med. 2010;152:1-9.

[61] Walker J, Robinson J, Stewart J, Jacob S. Does enteric-coated aspirin result in a lower incidence of gastrointestinal complications compared to normal aspirin? Interact Cardiovasc Thorac Surg. 2007 Aug;6(4):519-22.

[62] Yeomans N, Lanas A, Labenz J, van Zanten SV, van Rensburg C, Rácz I, Tchernev K, Karamanolis D, Roda E, Hawkey C, Nauclér E, Svedberg LE. Efficacy of esomeprazole (20 mg once daily) for reducing the risk of gastroduodenal ulcers associated with continuous use of low-dose aspirin. Am J Gastroenterol. 2008;103(10):2465-73.

[63] Straus WL, Ofman JJ, MacLean C, et al. Do NSAIDs cause dyspepsia? A meta-analysis evaluating alternative definitions. Am J Gastroenterol 2002 Aug;97(8):1951-8

[64] Alam T, Clyne CA, White CM. Pharmacologic and nonpharmacologic thromboprophylactic strategies in atrial fibrillation. J Comparative Effectiveness Res 2012;1(3): 225-39.

[65] Nakaji G, Fujihara M, Fukata M, Yasuda S, Odashiro K, Maruyama T, Akashi K. Influence of common cardiac drugs on gastroesophageal reflux disease: multicenter questionnaire survey. Int J Clin Pharmacol Ther. 2011;49(9):555-62.

[66] Watson DJ, Bolognese JA, Yu C, Krupa D, Curtis S. Use of gastroprotective agents and discontinuations due to dyspepsia with the selective cyclooxygenase-2 inhibitor etoricoxib compared with non-selective NSAIDs. Curr Med Res Opin. 2004;20(12): 1899-1908

[67] Coleman CI, Roberts MS, Sobieraj DM, Lee S, Alam T, Kaur R. Effect of dosing frequency on chronic cardiovascular disease medication adherence. Curr Med Res Opin. 2012;28(5):669-80.

[68] Chey WD, Wong BC; Practice Parameters Committee of the American College of Gastroenterology. American College of Gastroenterology guideline on the management of Helicobacter pylori infection. Am J Gastroenterol. 2007;102(8):1808-25.

[69] Li XQ, Andersson TB, Ahalström M, et al. Comparison of Inhibitory Effects of the Proton Pump-Inhibiting Drugs Omeprazole, Esomeprazole, Lansoprazole, Pantopra-

zole and Rabeprazole on Human Cytochrome P450 Activities. Drug Metab Dispo, 2004, 32(8):821-7.

[70] Ogilvie BW, Yerino P, Kazmi F, et al. The Proton Pump Inhibitor, Omeprazole, but not Lansoprazole or Pantoprazole, is a Metabolism-Dependent Inhibitor of CYP2C19: Implications for Coadministration With Clopidogrel. Drug Metab Dispos, 2011, 39(11):2020-33.

[71] Angiolillo DJ, Gibson CM, Cheng S, et al. Differential Effects of Omeprazole and Pantoprazole on the Pharmacodynamics and Pharmacokinetics of Clopidogrel in Healthy Subjects: Randomized, Placebo-Controlled, Crossover Comparison Studies. Clin Pharmacol Ther, 2011, 89(1):65-74.

[72] Siller-Matula JM, Spiel AO, Lang IM, et al. Effects of Pantoprazole and Esomeprazole on Platelet Inhibition by Clopidogrel. Am Heart J, 2009, 157(1):148.e1-5

[73] Juurlink DN, Gomes T, Ko DT, Szmitko PE, Austin PC, Tu JV, Henry DA, Kopp A, Mamdani MM. A population-based study of the drug interaction between proton pump inhibitors and clopidogrel. CMAJ. 2009;180(7):713-8.

[74] Kreutz RP, Stanek EJ, Aubert R, et al. Impact of Proton Pump Inhibitors on the Effectiveness of Clopidogrel After Coronary Stent Placement: The Clopidogrel Medco Outcomes Study. Pharmacotherapy, 2010, 30(8):787-96.

[75] Ho PM, Maddox TM, Wang L, et al. Risk of Adverse Outcomes Associated With Concomitant Use of Clopidogrel and Proton Pump Inhibitors Following Acute Coronary Syndrome. JAMA, 2009, 301(9):937-44.

[76] Pezalla E, Day D, and Pulliadath I. Initial Assessment of Clinical Impact of a Drug Interaction Between Clopidogrel and Proton Pump Inhibitors. J Am Coll Cardiol, 2008, 52(12):1038-9.

[77] O'Donoghue ML, Braunwald E, Antman EM, et al. Pharmacodynamic Effect and Clinical Efficacy of Clopidogrel and Prasugrel with or without a Proton-pump Inhibitor: an Analysis of two randomised trials. Lancet, 2009, 374(9694):989-97.

[78] Bhatt DL, Cryer BL, Contant CF, et al. Clopidogrel With or Without Omeprazole in Coronary Artery Disease. N Engl J Med, 2010, 363(20):1909-17.

[79] Abraham NS, Hlatky MA, Antman EM, et al. ACCF/ACG/AHA 2010 Expert Consensus Document on the Concomitant Use of Proton Pump Inhibitors and Thienopyridines: A Focused Update of the ACCF/ACG/AHA 2008 Expert Consensus Document on Reducing the Gastrointestinal Risks of Antiplatelet Therapy and NSAID Use: A Report of the American College of Cardiology Foundation Task Force on Expert Consensus Documents. Circulation 2010;122(24):2619-33.

[80] White CM, Song J, Kalus J. Cardiac Arrhythmias, Chapter 20. In: Alldredge BK, Corelli RL, Ernst ME (Eds). Applied Therapeutics: The Clinical Use of Drugs. 10th Edition. Lippincott Williams & Wilkins, NY, NY. 2012 pg. 20.1-20.35.

[81] Contreras F, Fouillioux C, Lares M, et al. Effects of metoclopramide and metoclopramide/dopamine on blood pressure and insulin release in normotensive, hypertensive, and type 2 diabetic subjects. Am J Therapeut 2010;17:320-4.

[82] Blanco M, Jelambi I, Perez G et al. The effect of intravenous metoclopramide on blood pressure in normotensive and hypertensive subjects. Int J Clin Pharmacol Ther 1996;34:390-2.

[83] Frankton S, Balthun S, Husain E, Davis K, Grossman AB. Phaeochromocytoma crisis presenting with profound hypoglycemia and subsequent hypertension. Hormones 2009;8:65-70.

[84] Guillemot J, Compagnon P, Cartier D, et al. Metoclopramide stimulates catecholamine- and granin-derived peptide secretion from pheochromocytoma cells through activation of serotonin type 4 (5-HT4) receptors. Endocrine-Related Cancer 2009;16:281-90.

[85] Freestone S, Duffield J, Lee MR. Pressor effect of metoclopramide in phaeochromocytoma. Postgrad Med J 1996;72:188-9.

[86] Fischer AA, Davis MW. Serotonin syndrome caused by selective serotonin reuptake-inhibitors-metoclopramide interaction. Ann Pharmacother 2002;36:67-71.

[87] Luchsinger A, Grilli M, Velasco M. Metoclopramide and domperidone block the antihypertensive effect of bromocriptine in hypertensive patients. Am J Therapeut 1998;5:81-8.

[88] Martin G, Forte P, Luchsinger A, et al. Dopamine-induced antihypertensive effects and plasma insulin are blocked by metoclopramide in labetolol-treated patients. J Clin Pharmacol 1994;34:91-4.

Chapter 9

Functional Gastrointestinal Symptoms in Women with Pelvic Endometriosis

Yves Muscat Baron

Additional information is available at the end of the chapter

http://dx.doi.org/10.5772/56611

1. Introduction

Gastrointestinal symptoms are frequently encountered in women diagnosed with endometriosis. Women with endometriosis appear to complain more commonly of gastrointestinal symptoms such as gastro-oesophageal reflux and dyspepsia. The psychological profile of patients with endometriosis may promote these symptoms. As a reaction to high levels of perceived stress, neuroendocrine-immune imbalance has been demonstrated in women diagnosed with endometriosis. Pharmacological agents used to treat psychological dysfunction, and symptoms of endometriosis such as dysmenorrhoea, may lead to undesirable gastrointestinal symptoms.

Through neuroendocrine and immunological intermediaries, the gastrointestinal system may also interact with the physiology of the female genital system. These variables have directed some workers to suggest an interrelationship between both systems including the occurrence of pathology. Gastrointestinal symptoms may act as a guide to dietary modification which may result in improvement in the symptomatology of endometriosis.

2. Epidemiology of gastrointestinal symptoms and endometriosis

It is becoming apparent that although anatomically separate, gastrointestinal symptoms do overlap with pelvic endometriosis. Endometriosis is the occurrence of endometrial tissue outside the uterus. Endometriotic deposits are mainly found on the ovaries, utero-sacral ligaments and pelvic peritoneum. Endometriosis affects one fourth of young women under the age of 30 years with an overall incidence of 7% to 10 % of women. Subfertility has been noted in 20-50% of women found to have endometriosis while more than 80% of women complaining of chronic pelvic pain have been diagnosed as having this condition. Conversely endometriosis has been diagnosed in 20-50% of women who were completely asymptomatic, unaware that they had this pelvic pathology [1].

Gastrointestinal symptoms appear more prevalent in women diagnosed with pelvic endometriosis [2,3,]. Specific signs and symptoms result in frequent medical consultation are associated with presence of endometriosis [4]. The anatomical separation between the gastrointestinal tract and the female genital tract may prima facie, appear disparate without any anatomical or physiological association. In a study by Muscat Baron et al [5,6] however, gastrointestinal symptoms such as heartburn and dyspepsia were significantly more commonly found in women with endometriosis as compared to a control group. This was a prospective trial involving 57 menstrual women who had undergone laparoscopic examination of the pelvis for a diverse number of abdominal and gynaecological symptoms. The women recruited to the study were asked a comprehensive questionnaire which included information on gastrointestinal symptoms, gynaecological symptoms, dietary intolerance and general symptoms. During laparoscopy 23 women were diagnosed as having pelvic endometriosis while in the other thirty-four this diagnosis was excluded. Upper gastrointestinal symptoms such as heartburn and dyspepsia were found more commonly in the endometriosis group reaching statistical significance ($p < 0.001$). These results posed the enquiry as to why two apparently anatomically distant systems, that is the gastrointestinal tract and the female reproductive system, should influence each other [5,6].

Women diagnosed with endometriosis have been shown to have concomitant irritable bowel syndrome symptoms. Ballard et al have shown that women with pelvic endometriosis were also diagnosed with irritable bowel syndrome (OR 1.6 [95% CI: 1.3-1.8]) [4]. Lower gastrointestinal symptoms in the form of diarrhoea and loose stools have been found more commonly found in women diagnosed with endometriosis. As opposed to the upper gastro-intestinal tract, both the small and to a greater extent the large bowel is in close proximity with the female genital tract. Both systems (intestinal and reproductive) throughout their physiological functioning are likely to influence each other [5,6].

It must be kept in mind that gastrointestinal symptoms commonly occur in the general population. Although estimates vary according to the diagnostic criteria used, 10–40% of the adult population experience heartburn and dyspepsia in Western countries. Gastro-oesophageal reflux disease increases with age, rising sharply beyond the fourth decade. More than half of the patients effected are aged between 45 and 64[7].

Dyspepsia also affects between 20% and 40% of the Western populations. A quarter of all cases of dyspepsia are though to be related to gastric and duodenal ulcers [8]. Several studies from the 1940's to the 1980's reported that population prevalence of 18%[9], 26%[10] and 31% [11] of people referred with dyspepsia were found to have peptic ulcers. Recently this percentage has fallen to around 10–15%[7]. Although mortality in people with gastrointestinal disorders is not raised compared with the general population, these disorders have a significant impact on quality of life. It has been shown that 75% of people with heartburn and dyspepsia suffered persistent symptoms and impaired quality of life over periods of 10 years or more; 30–50% never returned to work and were unable to carry out household tasks [12].

http://dx.doi.org/10.5772/56611

3. Pathogenesis of endometriosis and gastrointestinal symptoms

The enigmatic pathogenesis of endometriosis has led to the formulation of several hypotheses, but none have been proven conclusively. The elusiveness of its pathology has directed some workers to search beyond the female genital tract and concentrate their efforts at the gastrointestinal system, the small and large bowel being in close anatomical proximity to the female genital tract (Figure 1.)[5,6,13]. The overlap of symptoms between both the gastrointestinal pathology and endometriosis influences clinical practice and in several women leads to delayed or misdiagnosis (Figure 1.).

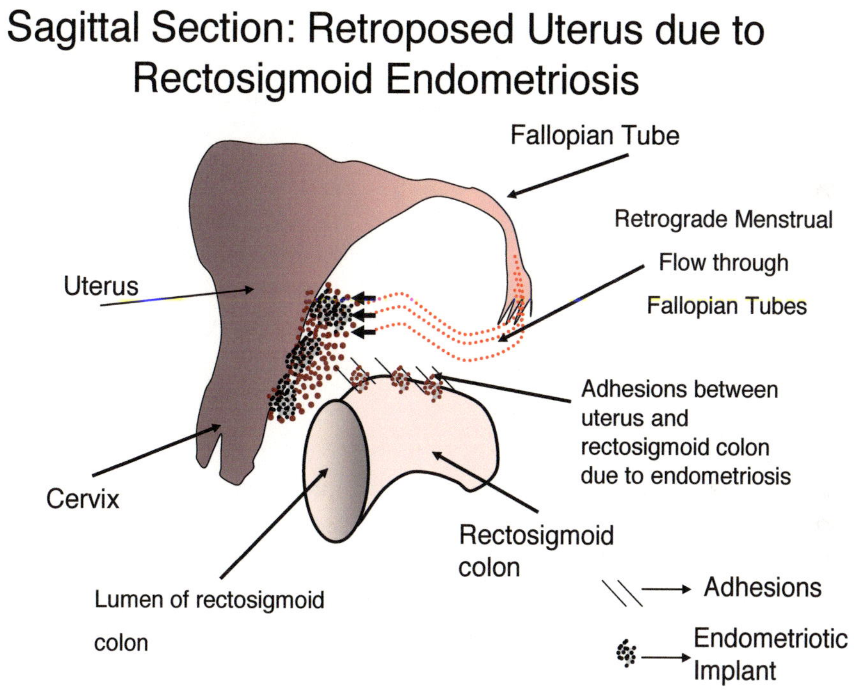

Figure 1. Following retrograde menstrual flow through the Fallopian tubes, endrometriotic deposits colonize adjacent peritoneal structures. The peritoneal structures involved include ovaries, utero-sacral ligaments and adjacent bowel especially the rectosigmoid colon. Following endometriotic deposition adhesion formation results. This may lead to a retroverted uterus due to endometriosis-included adhesions between rectosigmoid colon and posterior aspect of uterus, with obliteration of the Pouch of Douglas.

Physiological studies indicate that gastric emptying does not appear to be affected by the menstrual cycle. Abdominal symptoms related to the upper gastrointestinal tract appear more commonly during the follicular phase. During the follicular phase the transit time in the small bowel is longer. The normal menstrual cycle has no effect on gastric motility suggesting that gastric emptying does not change significantly between the follicular and luteal phases [14]. Almost 50% of women with irritable bowel syndrome report a perimenstrual increase in symptoms [15].

4. Psychological background to the co-existence of endometriosis and gastrointestinal symptoms

Emotional and mood disorders in women have been significantly detected in women suffering from endometriosis. These disorders were found more commonly in women with endometriosis (11/23 $p < 0.03$), admitting regular administration of anxiolytic and/or anti depressant therapy for symptoms related to significant anxiety or depression [5].

In a prospective study by [16], out of 104 women diagnosed with pelvic endometriosis 87.5% of women complained of anxiety. This anxiety state was mild in 24% and severe in 63.5% of the subjects studied. Correlations between pain intensity and anxiety symptoms, were also obtained using the State-Trait Anxiety Inventory (STAI) (state, P=0.009; trait, P=0.048) and the Hamilton Rating Scale for Anxiety (HAMA) (P=0.0001). Moreover anxiolytic treatment with benzodiazepines such as clonazepam has been used in women with endometriosis. A number of these subjects also required prolonged treatment with serotonin selective serotonin re-uptake inhibitors (SSRI's) [16].

Depression has also been noted to be prevalent in women with pelvic endometriosis, a high proportion of which require anti-depressant therapy. Depressive symptoms were observed in 86.5% of patients with pelvic endometriosis (mild in 22.1%, moderate in 31.7%, and severe in 32.7%) [16]. In a similar percentage (86%) of women, depression was detected in the women with endometriosis complaining of chronic pelvic pain [17]. Work inhibition, dissatisfaction, and sadness, were observed at a significantly higher rates in the group with abdominal pain [17]

The above mentioned psychological profile of these women may have been moulded from a very young age. The cyclical experience of the symptoms of severe dysmenorrhoea and menstrual disorders from puberty, may have conditioned these women to acquire certain personality traits as a reaction to the cyclical physical and subsequent psychological suffering they sustained [16]. Lower quality of life indices correlated with high pain scores. Lower quality of life status in psychological and environmental perspectives resulted in an inverse relationship between pain scores and the psychological dimension of quality of life ($r = -0.310$, $P = .02$)[18].

Mood disorders in adult women with endometriosis are associated with co-morbidities such as pain syndromes including irritable bowel syndrome, vulvodynia, fibromyalgia and asthma have been noted with in adult women with endometriosis. These co-morbidities appear to have their conception early in reproductive life in adolescents and young women. A study by Smorgick et al (2013) reviewing 138 adolescents/young women (younger than 24 years) demonstrated a prevalence of comorbid pain syndromes 56% women, mood conditions in 66 (48%) women, and asthma in 31 (26%) women [19].

Exacerbations of gastrointestinal motility disorders such as gastro-oesophageal reflux and irritable bowel syndrome are associated with the emergence of psychosocial stressors. Naliboff et al [20] assessed 60 subjects with current heartburn symptoms and correlated for the occurrence of stressful life events retrospectively over the preceding 6 months and prospectively for 4 months. The occurrence of a severe, sustained life stress during the previous 6 months significantly predicted increased heartburn symptoms during the following 4 months. Anxiety showed the strongest correlation to impaired quality of life and depression to heartburn medication use. Similar to other chronic conditions such as irritable bowel syndrome, heartburn severity appears to be most responsive to major life events. Both heartburn and irritable bowel syndrome may be related to gastrointestinal motility disorders[20]. In the upper gastrointestinal tract oesophageal acid exposure due to inhibition of gastric emptying of acid may lead to heartburn. Alternatively motility disorders affecting the lower intestinal tract lead to irritable bowel syndrome.

On further investigation of gynaecological complaints, once the diagnosis of endometriosis is established, the phobia of infertility may set in, further compounding the psychological profile. If infertility does occur in these women, then depressive symptoms are more likely to appear. Self-reported depression was more common in subfertile women (n = 1,031), with endometriosis (O.R. 5.43, C.I. 4.01-7.36) compared with fertile women (n = 4,905) [21].

5. Neuro-endocrine imbalance in association with Gastrointestinal symptoms and Endometriosis

The majority of women suffering from endometriosis are well versed in their condition. With easy access to medical literature, besides subfertility, the risk of inflammatory bowel disease and ovarian cancer has now become universally known to most women suffering from endometriosis [21]. All these factors exacerbate the tenuous emotional status of these women (Figure 2.)

In response to high levels of perceived stress, neuroendocrine-immune imbalance has been alluded to as a reaction to the symptoms of endometriosis. Serum prolactin levels were significantly higher in infertile women with stage III-IV endometriosis (28.9 +/- 2.1 ng/mL) than in healthy controls (13.2 +/- 2.1 ng/mL)[22]. Elevated serum cortisol levels were noted in infertile women with stage III-IV endometriosis (20.1 +/- 1.3 ng/mL) compared to controls (10.5 +/- 1.4 ng/mL) [22]. Perception of stress has been noted to trigger or intensify the incidence or exacerbation of diseases such as inflammatory bowel disease, immunological cutaneous conditions, or pregnancy complications such as spontaneous miscarriage and pre-eclampsia. The effect on the immunity of the intestinal mucosa by stress has been implicated as a potential mechanism leading to irritable bowel syndrome. This is thought to be mediated through altered function of the hypothalamic-pituitary-adrenal axis and the sympathetic nervous system. Both of these systems can modulate mucosal immune function. A study by Chang et al indicated that basal adrenocorticotropin hormone levels were significantly blunted ($P < 0.05$), while basal and stimulated plasma cortisol levels were higher in patients with irritable bowel syndrome. Patients with irritable bowel syndrome presenting with diarrhoea had significantly decreased mRNA expression of mucosal cytokines [interleukin (IL)-2, IL-6] in the sigmoid colon versus controls ($P < 0.05$) [24].

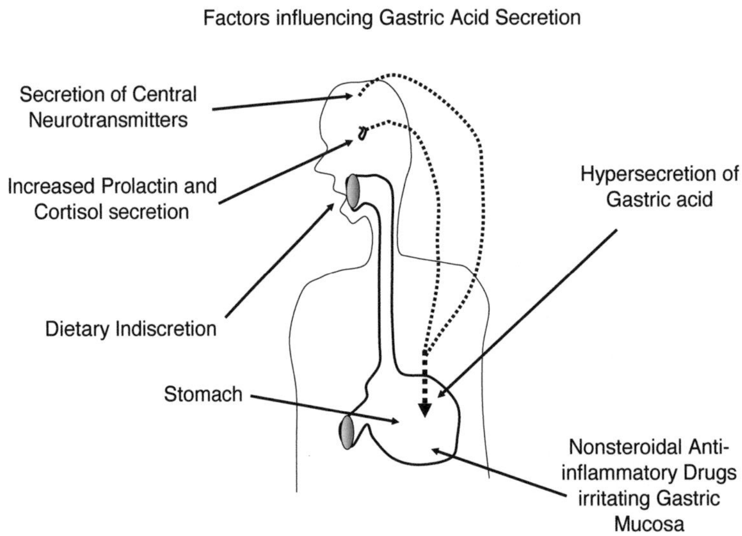

Figure 2. The secretion of central neurotransmitters and hormones such as cortisol and prolactin increase the secretion of gastric acid. This compounded by dietary indiscretion and injudicious ingestion of nonsteroidal inflammatory agents increase risk for gastric mucosal ulceration.

The association between psychological status and the gastrointestinal tract is well established. Dr William Beaumont in 1833 demonstrated the influence of psychological stress on gastric mucosal changes. Acclaimed as the Father of Gastric Physiology, Dr Beaumont carried out observations and experiments on an individual known as Alexis St Martin. St Martin had sustained a gastric fistula followed gunshot wound to the stomach, exposing a sliver of gastric mucosa. Beaumont observed that the exposed gastric mucosa instantly reddened when St Martin was angered, connecting the neuroendocrine-emotional status with gastric physiology [25].

Heartburn and dyspepsia are acknowledged symptoms related with psychological and mood disorders. Gastro-oesophageal reflux disease can be anatomically traced back to dysfunction of the gastro-oesophageal junction, however psychological factors can play an important role in the exacerbation of heart-burn. Well defined personality factors modulate the effect of stress on the gastro-oesophageal junction, just as they can influence the perception and assessment of symptoms. Gastric and small intestinal motor disorders and stomach acid hypersecretion, interact with psychological and neurohormonal resulting in the pathogenesis of dyspepsia. Greater proximal extension of acid during reflux episodes has been demonstrated in patients with proven gastro-oesophageal reflux disease. These patients describe a shorter history of symptom onset and worse anxiety scores. Endoscopic investigation depict findings compatible with gastritis [26].

Altered secretion of gastric acid in the stomach has been linked with a vast array of modulators supporting the neuro-endocrinological connection. Central neurotransmitters and/or neuromodulators may excite or inhibit gastric acid secretion. Excitatory neuro-endocrine modulators such as gamma-aminobutyric acid (GABA), acetylcholine, thyrotropin releasing hormone,

http://dx.doi.org/10.5772/56611

oxytocin have been cited. On the contrary, noradrenaline, adenosine, bombesin, calcitonin-gene related peptide, corticotropin releasing factor, beta-endorphin, neurotensin, neuropeptide Y, insulin-like growth factor II and prostaglandins have been shown to inhibit gastric acid secretion.

Several of these neuro-endocrine mediators have also been noted in endometriosis. Deep infiltrating endometriosis is associated with severe and frequent chronic pelvic pain. In these cases significantly more nerve fibres are detected histologically, than in superficial peritoneal endometriotic lesions. Deep infiltrating endometriotic lesions were shown to be innervated abundantly by sensory nerve fibres utilizing acetylcholine and norepinephrine as neurotransmitters [27]. Women with endometriosis have been noted to have lower levels of progesterone in serum in the follicular phase and progesterone levels were inversely correlated to pain scores. Progesterone receptor positive peritoneal lymphocytes of CD56(+) and CD8(+) type were increasing found in advanced endometriosis. Cytokine secretion by peritoneal cells, was higher in cells derived from endometriosis patients and could be further heightened by corticotrophin releasing hormone mediated inflammation. Peripheral corticotrophin releasing hormone increasing with anxiety and emotional stress, might contribute to the peritoneal inflammation present in endometriosis [28,29].

6. Gastrointestinal symptoms, the menstrual cycle and endometriosis

An increase in the prevalence of gastro-intestimal symptoms are noted around the time of menses and early menopause [30]. These are periods in the reproductive cycle whereby a significant decline or low level of ovarian hormones in serum are noted. These observations suggest that estrogen and progesterone withdrawal may contribute either directly or indirectly to the occurrence of gastrointestinal symptoms and possibly to pathology [30].

Due to significant overlap between the symptoms of endometriosis and symptoms related to endometriotic deposits on the gastrointestinal system, endometriosis has been referred to the great masquerader. Moreover the menstrual cycle may also impact on gastrointestinal function. As confirmed in the general literature, the presence of frequent menstruation in our study in patients with endometriosis increased the likelihood of related gastrointestinal symptoms.

Abdominal symptoms are significantly more pronounced at the beginning of the menstrual cycle in the follicular phase [14]. Around 30% of otherwise asymptomatic women may experience gastrointestinal symptoms at the time of menstruation, and almost fifty percent of women with irritable bowel syndrome complain of a perimenstrual increase in symptoms. Nausea, epigastric pain, and loose stools diarrhoea are more prevalent at the time of menses in women complaining of bowel dysfunction. Patients complaining of bowel motility symptoms indicate that stomach pain was higher throughout the menstrual cycle. Patients with endometriosis complained of cramping pain more commonly in the perimenstrual phase [31].

Intestinal motility disorders may be associated with the genesis of endometriosis and conversely endometriosis may influence intestinal motility. Preclinical studies have shown significantly more colonic damage, myeloperoxidase activity, and leucocyte count numbers than controls did. Increased tension in the longitudinal muscle correlated with leuccytosis and colonic damage. Mabrouk et al have shown that in deep infiltrating endometriosis, internal anal sphincter tone was increased in 20 of 25 patients. Responses to a defaecatory function questionnaire, indicated that incomplete evacuation was the most common symptom [32].

Premenstrual symptoms may be affected by dietary components. Soy products have not been shown to alter Moos Menstrual Distress scores significantly during premenstrual phase [33]. However the ingestion of total saturated and monounsaturated fats were significantly correlated with change in Moos Menstrual Distress scores which assesses a number of premenstrual and menstrual symptomatology and subscale 'pain' in the premenstrual phase after controlling for the covariates. The consumption of cereals/potatoes/starches was significantly inversely correlated with a change in total Moos Menstrual Distress scores in the premenstrual phase [33].

Presumably due to hormonal and menstrual differences twice as many women as men seek health services for irritable bowel syndrome as men. The presence of dyspepsia in women, was found to be a significant independent risk factor for new-onset irritable bowel syndrome ([OR] = 2.14; 95% CI, 1.56–2.94). The majority of women with irritable bowel syndrome requesting medical consultation are of reproductive age experiencing the hormonal fluctuations of the menstrual cycle. However, after the age of 50 most population surveys have reported a decline in the prevalence of irritable bowel syndrome[34]. Both oestrogen and progesterone influence 5-hydroxytryptamine, an amine which is known to effect intestinal motor-sensory function. During menstruation where oestrogen and progesterone levels reach their lowest levels in the menstrual cycle, the platelet-depleted plasma concentration of 5-hydroxytryptamine in irritable bowel syndrome patients with diarrhoea were similar to healthy controls [35]. Compared to males, females with irritable bowel syndrome more commonly display non-painful gastrointestinal symptoms, constipation and somatic discomfort. There appear to be different gender-related pathways in sympathetic nervous system responses to rectosigmoid stimulation. In a study by Chang et al 58 patients with irritable bowel syndrome underwent barostat-assisted distensions of the rectum and sigmoid colon. Women with irritable bowel syndrome had significantly lower rectal discomfort thresholds compared with men with irritable bowel syndrome and healthy women who were the least sensitive. There were no significant differences in rectal discomfort thresholds between men with irritable bowel syndrome and healthy men. In both irritable bowel syndrome and control groups, women demonstrated significantly lower discomfort thresholds after noxious sigmoid stimulation ($P<0.01$) compared to men. [36].

Oral contraception results in relatively strict regulation of the menstrual cycle. Moreover the use of oral contraception is associated with reduced menstrual loss and diminished levels of dysmenorrhoea. During menstruation, women with irritable bowel syndrome using oral contraceptives complain of less cognitive, anxiety, and depression symptoms ($p < 0.05$) but no differences were seen for most symptoms of irritable bowel syndrome [37]. There may be a differential effect of oral contraception depending on gastrointestinal symptom pattern.

http://dx.doi.org/10.5772/56611

The presentation of endometriosis may mimic that of inflammatory bowel disease. Cramping pain of dysmenorrhea is due to contraction of uterine smooth muscle under the influence of prostaglandins, released by the endometrium during menstruation. The inflammatory process in active inflammatory bowel disease is intimately related to prostaglandin levels. Elevated prostaglandin levels increase contractility of intestinal smooth muscle resulting in diarrhoea and abdominal pain.

There is critical importance in the clinical distinction between the diagnosis of endometriosis and inflammatory bowel disease. Nonsteroidal anti-inflammatory drugs are administered to relieve the symptoms of dysmenorrhoea in the presence and absence of endometriosis. However Nonsteroidal anti-inflammatory drugs are contraindicated in inflammatory bowel disease due to the risk of exacerbation of inflammatory bowel disease.

Dietary components in relation to symptomatic Endometriosis and Gastrointestinal symptoms

Psychological stress is also related to injudicious ingestion of dietary components that may irritate the gastrointestinal tract. Somatization, state and trait anxiety and binge eating are significant predictors of coexistent gastrointestinal disorders.

Nutrition research suggests that vitamins, minerals, and other dietary components are important underpinnings of general physical and mental health. Moreover, dietary modification may even be useful in treating mood disorder by providing a more favourable risk-benefit ratio than contemporary psychotropic agents [38].

The body mass index of women who experience depression is significantly higher than controls. Meta-analyses confirm a reciprocal link between depressive states and obesity. Self-confirmed depression, and clinically diagnosed depression are strongly associated with high body mass index.

6.1. Pharmacological treatment of endometriosis and gastrointestinal symptoms

Anxiety states have been shown to result in excessive ingestion of benzodiazepines, relaxing lower oesophageal sphincter pressure and subsequently facilitating gastro-oesophageal reflux. Depression treated with clomipramine was associated with an increased risk of oesophageal reflux (OR 4.6, 95% CI 2.0-10.6) in a duration- and dose-dependent manner [39].

Moreover, depression and its therapy were found to be predictive of developing obesity. Early during the first 6 weeks of nortriptyline treatment, weight gain commences, reaching on average 1.2 kg at 12 weeks with a resultant 0.44% increase in body mass index [40].

Chronic consumption of nonsteroidal anti-inflammatory agents to counter endometriosis-induced dysmenorrhoea and menorrhagia may lead to ulceration of the gastric mucosa. The degree of nonsteroidal anti-inflammatory gastropathy may be severe enough to develop gastric and duodenal ulceration. It appears that there is sufficient evidence to indicate that administration of nonsteroidal anti-inflammatory drugs could be considerably attenuated and adverse effects, avoided if medical practitioners were persuaded to change their prescribing practices [41].

7. Conclusion

There appears to be co-existence of gastrointestinal symptoms and endometriosis. The linkage between gastrointestinal symptoms and endometriosis may be due the psychological background and neuro-endocrine mediation. Gastrointestinal symptoms have been related to both dietary indiscretion and psychological stress both of which may, for a variety of reasons, be commonly encountered in women with endometriosis. Moreover treatment of the symptoms of endometriosis may aggravate gastrointestinal symptoms.

In suspected endometriosis, meticulous consultation carefully assessing the woman's symptomatology is required to avoid delay or possibly misdiagnosis. A delay or misdiagnosis may further exacerbate the psychological background of anxiety and depression, together with the incidence of gastrointestinal symptoms. The co-existence of gastrointestinal conditions and endometriosis may require a multi-disciplinary approach to enact effective treatment.

Author details

Yves Muscat Baron*

Address all correspondence to: yambaron@go.net.mt; yves.muscat.baron@gov.mt

Department of Obstetrics and Gynaecology, Mater Dei University Hospital, Msida, Malta

References

[1] Mounsey AL, Wilgus A, Slawson DC. Diagnosis and management of endometriosis. American Family Physician 2006;74:594-600.

[2] Roman H, Ness J, Suciu N, Bridoux V, Gourcerol G, Leroi AM, Tuech JJ, Ducrotté P, Savoye-Collet C, Savoye G. Are digestive symptoms in women presenting with pelvic endometriosis specific to lesion localizations? A preliminary prospective study. Hum Reprod. 2012 Dec;27(12):3440-9. doi: 10.1093/humrep/des322. Epub 2012 Sep 7.

[3] Zwas FR, Lyon DT. Endometriosis. An important condition in clinical gastroenterology, Dig Dis Sci. 1991 Mar;36(3):353-64.

[4] Ballard KD, Seaman HE, de Vries CS, Wright JT. Can symptomatology help in the diagnosis of endometriosis? Findings from a national case-control study--Part 1. British Journal of Obstetrics and Gynaecology 2008; 5:1382-91.

[5] Muscat Baron Y, Dingli M, Camilleri Agius R, Brincat M. Gastrointestinal symptoms and dietary intolerance in women with endometriosis. Journal of Endometriosis 2011; 3: 99 – 104

[6] Muscat Baron Y, Dingli M, Camilleri Agius R, Brincat M. Endometriosis and Dietary Intolerance – a Connection. Journal of Italian Obstetrics and Gynaecology 2012; 1: 252 – 256.

[7] Kang JY. Systematic review: geographical and ethnic differences in gastro-oesophageal reflux disease. Aliment Pharmacology Therapeutics 2004; 20: 705-17.

[8] Grainger S L, Klass H J, Rake M O. et al. Prevalence of dyspepsia: the epidemiology of overlapping symptoms. Postgrad Med J 1994. 70154–161.161.

[9] Doll R, Avery Jones F, Buckatzsch M M. Occupational factors in the aetiology of gastric and duodenal ulcers, with an estimate of their incidence in the general population. London: HMSO, 1951

[10] Weir R D, Backett E M. Studies of the epidemiology of peptic ulcer in a rural community: prevalence and natural history of dyspepsia and peptic ulcer. Gut 1968; 975:83-84.

[11] Jones R H, Lydeard S. Prevalence of symptoms of dyspepsia in the community. BMJ 1989;298:31-.32.

[12] Gill D, Mayou R, Dawes M. et al Presentation, management and course of angina and suspected angina in primary care. J Psychosom Res 1999; 46349–358.358.

[13] Parazzini F, Chiaffarino F, Surace M, Chatenoud L, Cipriani S, Chiantera V, Benzi G, Fedele L. Selected food intake and risk of endometriosis. A prospective study of dietary fat consumption and endometriosis risk. Human Reproduction 2004; 19: 1755-9.

[14] Björnsson B, Orvar KB, Theodórs A, Kjeld M. The relationship of gastrointestinal symptoms and menstrual cycle phase in young healthy women. Laeknabladid 2008;2:677-82.

[15] Moore J, Barlow D, Jewell D, Kennedy S. Do gastrointestinal symptoms vary with the menstrual cycle? Br J Obstet Gynaecol. 1998 Dec;105(12):1322-5.

[16] Sepulcri R de P, do Amaral VF. Depressive symptoms, anxiety, and quality of life in women with pelvic endometriosis. European Journal Obstetric Gynecological Reproductive Biology 2009;42:-6.

[17] Lorençatto C, Petta CA, Navarro MJ, Bahamondes L, Matos A. Depression in women with endometriosis with and without chronic pelvic pain. Acta Obstetrica Gynecologia Scandinavica 2006;5:88-92.

[18] Souza C, Oliveira L, Scheffel C, Genro V, Rosa V, Chaves M, Cunha Filho J. Quality of life associated to chronic pelvic pain is independent of endometriosis diagnosis-a cross-sectional survey. Health Quality Life Outcomes 2011;9: 41.

[19] Smorgick N, Marsh CA, As-Sanie S, Smith YR, Quint EH. Prevalence of Pain Syndromes, Mood Conditions, and Asthma in Adolescents and Young Women with En-

dometriosis. Pediatr Adolesc Gynecol. 2013: S1083-3188(13)00002-8. [Epub ahead of print].

[20] Naliboff BD, Mayer M, Fass R, Fitzgerald LZ, Chang L, Bolus R, Mayer E. The effect of life stress on symptoms of heartburn. Psychosom Med 2004;66(3):426-34.

[21] Herbert DL, Lucke JC, Dobson AJ. Depression: an emotional obstacle to seeking medical advice for infertility. Fertility Sterility 2010;94:1817-21.

[22] Jess T, Frisch M, Tore K, Bo JK, Pedersen V, Nielsen M. Increased risk of inflammatory bowel disease in women with endometriosis: a nationwide Danish cohort study. Gut 2011;30:1095.

[23] Lima A P, Moura M D, Rosae SilvaA A. Prolactin and cortisol levels in women with endometriosis. Brazilian Journal Medical and Biological Research 2006; 39:1121-7.

[24] Chang L, Sundaresh S, Elliott J, et al. Dysregulation of the hypothalamic-pituitary-adrenal axis in irritable bowel syndrome. Neurogastroenterol Motil. 2009;21(2): 149-59.

[25] Beaumont W, 1833. Experiments and observations on the gastric juice and the physiology of digestion. Plattsburgh, PA: Printed by F. P. Allen.

[26] Shapiro M, Simantov R, Yair M, Leitman M, Blatt A, Scapa E, Broide E. Comparison of central and intraesophageal factors between gastroesophageal reflux disease (GERD) patients and those with GERD-related noncardiac chest pain. Disease Esophagus 2012; 10: 1442-2050.

[27] Wang G, Tokushige N, Markham R, Fraser IS. Rich innervation of deep infiltrating endometriosis. Human Reproduction 2009;24:827-34.

[28] Tariverdian N, Rücke M, Szekeres-Bartho J, Blois SM, Karpf EF, Sedlmayr P, Klapp BF, Kentenich H, Siedentopf F, Arck PC. Neuroendocrine circuitry and endometriosis: progesterone derivative dampens corticotropin-releasing hormone-induced inflammation by peritoneal cells in vitro. J Mol Med. 2010;88(3):267-78

[29] Tariverdian N, Theoharides TC, Siedentopf F, Gutiérrez G, Jeschke U, Rabinovich GA, Blois SM, Arck PC. Neuroendocrine-immune disequilibrium and endometriosis: an interdisciplinary approach. Semin Immunopathol. 2007 ;29(2):193-210.

[30] Hungin AP, Chang L, Locke GR, et al. Irritable bowel syndrome in the United States: Prevalence, symptom patterns and impact. Aliment Pharmacol Ther. 2005;21:1365–1375.

[31] Heitkemper M, and Chang L. Do Fluctuations in Ovarian Hormones Affect Gastrointestinal Symptoms in Women With Irritable Bowel Syndrome? Gend Med. 2009; 6(Suppl 2): 152–167

[32] Heitkemper MM, Cain KC, Jarrett ME, Burr RL, Hertig V, Bond EF,. Symptoms across the menstrual cycle in women with irritable bowel syndrome. American Journal of Gastroenterology 2003;98: 420-30.

[33] Mabrouk M, Ferrini G, Montanari G, Di Donato N, Raimondo D, Stanghellini V, Corinaldesi R, Seracchioli R. Does colorectal endometriosis alter intestinal functions? A prospective manometric and questionnaire-based study. Fertility Sterility 2012; 97:652-6.

[34] Nagata C, Hirokawa K, Shimizu N, Shimizu. Soy, fat and other dietary factors in relation to premenstrual symptoms in Japanese women. British Journal of Obstetrics and Gynaecology 2004; 111: 594-9.

[35] Lovell RM, Ford AC. Global prevalence of and risk factors for irritable bowel syndrome: a meta-analysis. Clin Gastroenterol Hepatol. 2012;10:712-721.

[36] Houghton LA, Brown H, Atkinson et al. 5-hydroxytryptamine signalling in irritable bowel syndrome with diarrhoea: effects of gender and menstrual status. Aliment Pharmacol Ther. 2009 ;30(9):919-29.

[37] Chang L, Mayer EA, Labus JS, Schmulson M, Lee OY, Olivas TI, Stains J, Naliboff BD. Effect of sex on perception of rectosigmoid stimuli in irritable bowel syndrome. Am J Physiol Regul Integr Comp Physiol. 2006;291(2):R277-84.

[38] Mayer EA, Berman S, Chang L, Naliboff BD. Sex-based differences in gastrointestinal pain. Eur J Pain. 2004 Oct;8(5):451-63.

[39] Frazier EA, Fristad MA, Arnold LE. Multinutrient supplement as treatment: literature review and case report of a 12-year-old boy with bipolar disorder. J Child Adolescent Psychopharmacology 2009;19: 453-60.

[40] van Soest EM, Dieleman JP, Siersema PD, Schoof L, Sturkenboom MC, Kuipers EJ. Tricyclic antidepressants and the risk of reflux esophagitis. American Journal Gastroenterology 2007; 102: 1870-7.

[41] Uher R, Mors O, Hauser J, et al,. Changes in body weight during pharmacological treatment of depression. International Neuropsychopharmacology 2011;14:367-75.

[42] Bloor K, Maynard A. Is there scope for improving the cost-effective prescribing of nonsteroidal anti-inflammatory drugs? Pharmacoeconomics 1996;9: 484-96.

Chapter 10

Dyspepsia and Opioid–Induced Bowel Dysfunction: The Role of Opioid Receptor Antagonists

Wojciech Leppert

Additional information is available at the end of the chapter

http://dx.doi.org/10.5772/56624

1. Introduction

Opioid analgesics are commonly and in most cases effectively used to manage chronic pain of moderate to severe intensity. Apart from analgesia, opioids exert numerous adverse effects, several of which impact the gastrointestinal (GI) tract. The chronic use of opioid analgesics in fact is commonly associated with adverse effects on the gastrointestinal tract. [1] Opioid–induced bowel dysfunction (OIBD) comprises gastrointestinal symptoms such as dry mouth, anorexia, gastroesophageal reflux (GERD), delayed digestion, abdominal pain, flatulence, bloating, nausea, vomiting, and constipation with hard stool and incomplete evacuation. Further, side effects from long–term opioid therapy may result in more serious intestinal complications such as faecal impaction with overflow diarrhea and incontinence, pseudo–obstruction (causing anorexia, nausea and vomiting), disturbance of drug absorption, and urinary retention and incontinence. OIBD may also lead to inappropriate opioid dosing and in consequence, insufficient analgesia. As a result, OIBD significantly deteriorate patients' quality of life and compliance with their treatment. Approximately one-third of patients treated with opioid analgesics do not adhere to the prescribed opioid regimen or simply quit the treatment due to OIBD symptoms [2].

Several strategies have been advocated to prevent or treat OIBD. Use of traditional laxatives is limited by their effectiveness, yet conveys their own adverse effects. Other possibilities comprise an opioid switch or changing the opioid administration route. New therapies now target opioid receptors in the gut as they represent a main source of OIBD symptoms. A combination of an opioid and opioid antagonist (oxycodone/naloxone) in prolonged release tablets and purely peripherally acting opioid receptor antagonist (methylnaltrexone) available in subcutaneous injections are currently available treatment options. This chapter reviews the pathophysiological basis and possible treatment strategies for OIBD.

2. Pathophysiological mechanism of opioid–induced bowel dysfunction

Opioids produce widespread effects throughout the gastrointestinal tract though several central and peripheral mechanisms. Such effects are a mixture of inhibitory and excitatory actions. Opioid peptides and their receptors are found throughout the gastrointestinal tract, especially in the gastric antrum and proximal duodenum. The basis for OIBD is therefore complex. The peripheral opioid effect on μ–opioid receptors in the gut wall likely plays a major role, but central effects may also be important [3]. μ–opioid receptors at a high density reside in neurons of myenteric and submucosal plexus and immune cells in the lamina propria [4]. Opioid receptors (predominantly μ, also κ and δ) are located in the gut wall in the myenteric plexus and in the submucosal plexus. The former are responsible for gut motility and the latter for secretion. These μ–opioid receptors are activated in the wall of the stomach, small and large intestine by both endogenous (e.g. enkephalins, endorphins and dynorphins) and exogenous (e.g. morphine, oxycodone, methadone) opioids and modify gastrointestinal function. Activation of μ–opioid receptors inhibits excitatory and inhibitory neural pathways within the enteric nervous system that coordinates motility. Inhibition of excitatory neural pathways depresses peristaltic contractions. On the other hand, the blockade of inhibitory neural pathways increases gut muscle activity, elevates resting muscle tone, and results in spasm and non–propulsive motility patterns. These mechanisms give rise to delayed gastric emptying and slowed intestinal transit [5].

Activation of opioid receptors in the submucosa inhibits water and electrolyte secretion into the gut lumen and increases fluid absorption from the intestine and accelerates blood flow in the gut wall [6]. Opioids increase activity in the sympathetic nervous system and thereby decrease secretion. Endocrine cells located in the epithelium also may play a role in regulating motor activity and secretion in the gut. Interms of motility, peripheral μ–opioid receptors inhibit intestinal transit independent of central μ–opioid receptors [7]. Moreover, opioids increase ileocaecal and anal sphincter tones and impair defecation reflex through reduced sensitivity to distension and increased internal anal sphincter tone [8]. Morphine administration leads to sphincter contraction and to a decreased emptying of pancreatic juice and bile [9], which may impair digestion. The anal sphincter dysfunction is an important factor in the sensation of anal blockage [10,11].

The central mechanism of opioid effects on the gastrointestinal tract is supported by the results of animal studies in which intracerebroventricular administration of morphine inhibited GI propulsion [12]. This effect was reversed by intracerebroventricular administration of naloxone [13] and vagotomy [14]. Intrathecal administration of morphine reduced gastroduodenal motility while intramuscular morphine gave additional effects. Thus, it seems that both central and peripheral opioid effects play a role in opioid GI effects [15]. The indirect evidence of both central and peripheral components of opioid effects on bowel function may be the observed 50–60% response rate to the treatment of OIBD with methylnaltrexone (MNTX), which displays only peripheral μ–opioid receptor antagonist effect in the treatment of patients with OIBD [16,17]. The stool remains in the gut lumen for a longer time, allowing greater absorption of fluid. Enhanced absorption combined with opioid inhibition

http://dx.doi.org/10.5772/56624

of secretomotor neurons in the epithelium of the gut [18] leads to the stool becomes hard and dry. In summary, OIBD is the consequence of reduced gastrointestinal motility, increased absorption of fluids from the gut and decreased epithelial secretion.

3. Dyspepsia

Dysfunction of the upper gastrointestinal tract (esophagus, stomach and duodenum) often manifests as dyspepsia. Dyspepsia represents a constellation of symptoms rather than a single disease entity. Its diverse symptoms may be expressed as epigastric pain, anorexia, belching, heartburn, bloating, nausea and vomiting, post–prandial fullness, early satiety, and/or regurgitation [19].

Two types of dyspepsia may be diagnosed:

- *Structural* (*organic*) *dyspepsia* for which a structural change can be demonstrated, often due to acid–related disease such as a gastric ulcer. In advanced cancer patients, symptoms may arise from NSAID, corticosteroid and bisphosphonate administration.
- *Functional dysmotility* (*non–ulcer dyspepsia*) due to dysmotility and/or altered sensitivity of the upper GI tract affecting the esophagus, stomach and duodenum. Esophageal and gastroduodenal dysmotility can be differentiated.

In cancer patients, it may be iatrogenic (e.g.; opioid–induced delayed gastric emptying) and associated with disease-related complications like hepatomegaly or massive ascites. Furthermore, paraneoplastic visceral autonomic neuropathy seems to play an important role. Opioids and other drugs such as anticholinergics, tricyclic antidepressants, benzodiazepines, nitrates and calcium channel blockers may decrease lower esophageal sphincter tone and lead to reflux (GERD) that would be aggravated secondarily by delayed gastric emptying. Gastric secretory and motor activity may be also affected by chronic alcoholism, diabetes, uremia, anxiety and depression. Gastroparesis is a symptomatic chronic disorder characterized by impaired gastric emptying in the absence of a structural cause. This occurs as a component of paraneoplastic syndromes, most commonly in the course of small cell lung, breast, ovarian cancer, Hodgkin disease or multiple myeloma. In addition to opioid adversely affecting gastric emptying, other drugs such as anticholinergics, neuroleptics or tricyclic antidepressants can aggravate gastroparesis. Meanwhile, concurrent conditions such as diabetes, prior gastric surgery, and neuromuscular disorders may further impair gastric emptying. Lastly, gastric or pancreatic tumors can inflict a mechanical outlet obstruction.

Another component that might co-exist is gastroesophageal reflux disease (GERD) due to reflux of gastric contents into the esophagus, causing mucosal damage and heartburn.

The prevalence of functional dyspepsia is high in the normal population (24–34%) and even higher in cancer patients (70%) [20]. Opioids adversely affect the esophagus. This class of drugs impairs esophageal inhibitory innervation and so induces spastic esophageal dysfunction while impairing lower esophageal relaxation, leading to swallowing difficulties (dysphagia). Opioids also reduce the lower esophageal sphincter (LES) pressure, thereby decreasing the barrier pressure between the stomach and the esophagus, producing acid-reflux symptoms. This effect is reversed by naloxone. Opioids inhibit gastric emptying, a product of enhanced gastric relaxation and heightened pyloric tone. This decrease in gastric emptying results from both central and peripheral effects, although a peripheral μ–opioid receptor mechanism is dominant. Opioid administration increases duodenal motility by generating patterns of contractions resembling migrating motor complex (MMC) phase III patterns. Endorphins in humans decrease antral phasic pressure activity and increase pyloric phasic pressure activity and induce MMC III–like bursts of contractile activity in the proximal gut followed by motor quiescence. Exogenous and endogenous opioids impair gastric emptying [21, 22].

The evaluation of patients with functional dyspepsia and gastroparesis is based on a careful history taking and physical examination that allow differentiating between functional and structural dyspepsia and GERD. The symptoms of gastroparesis, as quantified by the Gastroparesis Cardinal Symptom Index (GCSI), consists of 9 symptoms, each graded from 0 (none) to 5 (very severe), divided into 3 subscales: postprandial fullness/early satiety, nausea/vomiting, and bloating [23]. Upper endoscopy is usually needed to exclude mechanical obstruction and to assess for mucosal lesions. It is recommended in patients with alarming symptoms e.g.; those suspected for gastrointestinal bleeding. Endoscopy may be also conducted when symptoms develop with NSAIDs administration and when treatment with antisecretory drugs or antacids is unsuccessful. Blood tests assessing complete blood count and biochemistry might be useful. An ultrasound or CT abdominal scan is helpful to assess for cancer spread. In some patients, solid phase gastric scintigraphic emptying studies or breath tests may be needed to confirm gastroparesis. Other investigations such as electrogastrography, antroduodenal manometry are infrequently used in cancer patients.

4. Management of opioid–induced bowel dysfunction

4.1. The management of dyspepsia

a. Non–pharmacological measures

Treatment should be directed at cause of symptoms. Functional dyspepsia may be treated with non–pharmacological measures and drugs. The former comprise explanation and education of patients and families. Advice on the diet may play an important role. Fatty foods should be avoided as lipids impair gastric emptying, while lipids entering the duodenum may aggravate impaired gastric accommodation and gastric hypersensitivity. Medications that may cause dyspepsia (e.g. NSAIDs) should be discontinued when possible [24].

b. Pharmacological approach

Pharmacological treatment is usually needed. First-line therapy for dyspepsia is usually acid suppression. Proton pomp inhibitors (PPIs) such as omeprazole, esomeprazole or pantoprazole are used once daily in doses 20–40 mg, best given 30 minutes before breakfast. In cancer patients, prokinetic agents are commonly administered, aiming to counteract opioid–induced motility disorders.

Typically, metoclopramide is prescribed (commonly as 10 mg t.i.d.) for patients with functional dyspepsia, especially when symptoms arise from gastroparesis. Metoclopramide works mostly in the upper GI tract through blocking dopaminergic receptors. As metoclopramide also acts centrally, its use is associated with the added risk of extra–pyramidal effects, particularly in younger patients and children. Metoclopramide also inhibits the cytochrome, CYP2D6 enzyme [25]. The most common adverse effects of metoclopramide are restlessness, drowsiness and fatigue. Concomitant use of antidepressants, such as tricyclics, selective serotonin reuptake inhibitors (SSRIs) and newer serotonin–noradrenalin reuptake inhibitors (venlafaxine, duloxetine), may aggravate the adverse effects of metoclopramide [26]. Extrapyramidal effects are unlikely to occur when using domperidone, which does not cross blood–brain barrier [27]. Cisapride is a $5HT_4$ receptor agonist, affecting the entire GI tract; however, its cardiotoxicity has limited use [28].

Itopride works through peripheral blocking dopaminergic receptors. It inhibits acetylcholinesterase and so increases acetylcholine levels. Itopride works through the whole GI tract. It is devoid of activity at $5–HT_4$ and $5–HT_3$ receptors. Itopride is metabolized through monooxidase system. Thus, it has no significant risk of pharmacokinetic interactions with other drugs. Itopride does not cross blood–brain barrier and in consequence does not induce extrapyramidal effects. The dose usually equals 50 mg t. i. d. [29]

Prucalopride, a new prokinetic agent, is a highly selective $5HT_4$ receptor agonist that stimulates gut motility *in vitro* and *in vivo*. Prucalopride at 2–4 mg daily accelerates whole gut, gastric, small bowel and colonic transit in constipated patients [30]. The recommended dose is 1–2 mg once daily. Prucalopride is used in managing chronic constipation predominantly in women, but has not been evaluated in gastroparesis as yet [31]. Treatment is usually well-tolerated; typical adverse effects are headaches (present in 25–30% of treated patients), nausea (12–24%), abdominal pain or cramps (16–23%) and diarrhea (12–19%) [32]. Both itopride and prucapolpride appear safe relative to cardiac function.

Linaclotide is a minimally absorbed peptide guanylate cyclase-C agonist that appears quite effective for chronic constipation and the irritable bowel syndrome [33,34]. It looks promising in the treatment of gastroparesis and so may have a role in OBID.

Lubiprostone, a bicyclic fatty acid derived from prostaglandin E1, acts by specifically activating chloride channels on the apical aspect of gastrointestinal epithelial cells, producing a chloride-rich fluid secretion. These secretions soften the stool, increase intestinal motility, and so promote spontaneous bowel movements. Lubiprostone thus has value in treating functional constipation.

4.2. Oral and rectal laxatives for Opioid-induced Bowel Dysfunction

General measures to be taken in patients with OIBD and OIC include the assessment and applying prophylactic measures matched to the patient's general condition [35]. Change of diet (increased food and fluid intake), more physical activity, assuming a sitting position during bowel movement and obtaining privacy during defecation process are recommended [36]. Patients treated with opioids should be considered for prokinetic administration [37]. Any reversible causes such as hypercalcaemia should also be treated. Discontinuing or decreasing doses of drugs that may aggravate constipation (e.g. tricyclics, neuroleptics, anticholinergics) should also be considered. Patients and families should be educated about the means to prevent and treat OIBD [9].

In most patients with OIBD, laxatives are necessary. The general recommendation is to combine orally administered osmotic agents – usually lactulose or macrogol (PEG – polyethylene glycol) which have an osmotic effect in the colon [10] with stimulants activating on neurons in the myenteric and submucosal plexus in colon and reducing absorption of water and electrolytes from the intraluminal contents: anthracenes (senna), polyphenolics (bisacodyl) or sodium picosulphate. Unfortunately, these drugs exhibit limited efficacy in patients suffering from OIBD. Moreover, they may cause several adverse effects and must be administered on a regular basis [38]. Other classes of laxatives are faecal lubricants (liquid paraffin), stool softeners (surfactants: sodium docusate); however, they are usually ineffective when administered alone [39]. The use of bulk–forming agents such as fibre, bran, methylcellulose and psyllium seeds has limited role in patients with advanced constipation and warrant ingesting adequate fluids (at least 2 liters per day) [40–42]. Castor oil is not recommended due to its sudden stimulating effect on bowel motility and the risk of developing severe abdominal cramps [43]. If oral laxatives are found to be ineffective, rectal treatment should be considered.

Rectal laxatives comprise suppositories increasing intestinal motility through direct stimulation of the nerve endings in the myenteric ganglia of the colon, thus inducing peristalsis (bisacodyl) or using osmotic drugs (glycerol), which act by irritating the rectal mucosa and also enhance the colonic motility that subsequently triggers the defecation reflex. The next step if these agents prove ineffective is rectal enemas, either as normal saline (100–200 ml) or phosphates (120–150 ml).

The management of faecal impaction depends on the severity of symptoms (rectal pain, abdominal colicky pain, protruding hard faeces and faecal leakage). If the symptoms are not severe in case of soft faeces, administer bisacodyl 10–20 mg once daily either rectally or orally until bowel movements are achieved. If hard faeces are present, use glycerol and bisacodyl suppositories or osmotic enemas. Enemas of arachis oil (130 ml) or of decussate sodium (100 ml) followed by a phosphate enema next day may be appropriate. Macrogol (PEG) reduces the need for digital disimpaction. Digital stool evacuation may be necessary in cases of severe symptoms, when neither oral nor rectal treatment gives a desired effect and faecal impaction is not relieved, causing significant distress to the patient. As the procedure is quite painful and distressing, it should be performed with great caution and only when necessary and sometimes necessitating intravenous sedation with midazolam combined with opioids plus topical analgesics [44].

Polyethylene glycol (PEG) and sodium picosulphate are more effective than lactulose in OIC in cancer pain patients [45]. PEG specifically appears to be more effective than lactulose in

http://dx.doi.org/10.5772/56624

terms of weekly bowel movement frequency, patient satisfaction, ease of defecation and reduced constipation symptoms with similar treatment tolerance and slightly higher lactulose costs [46]. For palliative care patients, different laxative regimens have no real differences. Overall, there is limited efficacy of traditional laxatives; well-done randomised controlled trials are lacking [47].

4.3. Opioid switch

The possibility of opioid switch for OIBD should be considered as one of the available treatment options. Opioids, which seem to be more often associated with constipation, are codeine and dihydrocodeine (opioids for mild to moderate pain), morphine, oxycodone and hydromorphone (opioids for moderate to severe pain). These opioids may be switched to other opioids belonging to the same group but having less constipating effect: codeine or dihydrocodeine may be switched to tramadol; morphine, oxycodone or hydromorphone to transdermal opioids (fentanyl, buprenorphine) or to methadone [48,49]. The most convincing evidence supporting the benefits of the opioid switch as regards constipation relief comes from the morphine to transdermal fentanyl switch [50–53]. In contrast to clinical studies, observational surveys do not provide evidence for advantages of transdermal fentanyl over other opioid analgesics with respect to bowel function. [54-55] Other studies report similar or less intense constipating effects with transdermal buprenorphine compared to CR morphine [56] and after a switch from morphine to methadone [57–59]. There may be a benefit to administering tramadol rather than small morphine doses [60–62] or dihydrocodeine [63] with respect to the constipation intensity. However, no differences were found in constipation in cancer patients with pain between transdermal opioids (buprenorphine and fentanyl) and oral controlled release hydromorphone [64].

4.4. Targeted treatment of opioid–induced bowel dysfunction

Few clinical studies compared the efficacy of different laxatives [65] and controlled studies are lacking [66]. Certainly traditional laxatives do not target the cause of OIBD, which is predominantly associated with opioid analgesics binding and activating μ–opioid receptors in the GI tract [67]. Treatment directed at the cause of OIBD involves either using a combination of opioid analgesics with opioid receptor antagonists, which act both centrally and peripherally, or administering opioid receptor antagonists, which act exclusively peripherally. An important advantage of this approach is the fact that it is targeted treatment of OIBD and that it may be combined with oral laxatives, if necessary. Finally, this approach may eliminate the need for rectal measures, which patients tolerate poorly.

Apart from opioid antagonists with exclusively peripheral effects, opioid receptor antagonists with a central mode of action are naloxone, naltrexone and nalmefene. The majority of studies performed so far have used immediate release formulation of oral naloxone (IR naloxone). In spite of high IR naloxone efficacy in the treatment of OIBD, some patients experience opioid withdrawal symptoms and attenuation of analgesia, rendering IR naloxone less useful when administered alone [68–70]. Nalmefene [71] and nalmefene glucuronide [72] behave similarly.

4.5. Combined opioid receptor agonist with its antagonist

One of methods to decrease the frequency of constipation in patients requiring strong opioids is using formulation composed of an opioid and opioid receptor antagonist. The formulation combining oxycodone and naloxone is available in the form of prolonged release (PR) tablets containing both drugs in the ratio of 2:1 (PR oxycodone/PR naloxone 5 mg/2.5 mg, 10 mg/5 mg, 20 mg/10 mg, 40 mg/20 mg) [73]. The optimal 2:1 ratio of PR oxycodone/PR naloxone tablets was demonstrated in a phase II study rendering effective analgesia and improvement in bowel function with good treatment toleration in patients with severe chronic pain [74]. PR oxycodone/PR naloxone is registered for the indication of severe pain, which may only be successfully treated with opioid analgesics. In this formulation, naloxone counteracts the development of OIBD through inhibition of oxycodone effect on opioid receptors in the gut wall [75]. The starting PR oxycodone/PR naloxone doses in opioid–naive patients is 5 mg/2.5 mg b.i.d. Patients unsuccessfully treated with opioids for mild to moderate pain (tramadol, codeine, dihydrocodeine) may start with the dose 10 mg/5 mg b.i.d. When rotating from other opioids for moderate to severe pain to PR oxycodone/PR naloxone, the starting dose is established individually depending on the amount of previously administered opioid, analgesia and adverse effects. The maximal daily dose of PR oxycodone/PR naloxone recommended equals 40 mg/ 20 mg twice daily. However, in a study conducted in cancer patients with pain higher daily doses up to 120 mg/60 mg were effective and well–tolerated while symptoms of OIBD were decreased, compared to PR oxycodone administered alone [76].

Following oral administration, oxycodone displays high bioavailability (60 – 87%) and provides effective analgesia [77,78]. Naloxone exhibits low bioavailability after oral administration (< 2%) and undergoes extensive first–pass metabolism in the liver with the formation of naloxone–3–glucuronide [79]. Analgesic effect is not reversed by naloxone and no symptoms of opioid withdrawal occur. This effect of orally administered naloxone depends on normal liver function. Thus, any hepatic impairment should be carefully considered. In patients suffering from decompensated liver disease, PR oxycodone/PR naloxone administration is not recommended. There is a clinically observed difference between the administration of IR and PR formulations of naloxone. IR naloxone in some patients may attenuate analgesia or induce opioid withdrawal symptoms. The PR naloxone formulation prevents saturation of hepatic enzyme system responsible for naloxone metabolism and reduces the risk of opioid antagonism in the CNS [3].

PR oxycodone/PR naloxone provides similar analgesic efficacy to oxycodone with improvement in bowel function, a lower consumption of laxatives and more frequent spontaneous bowel movements [82]. during treatment with PR oxycodone/PR naloxone in comparison to PR oxycodone therapy [80–82]. Long–term therapy (up to 52 weeks) with PR oxycodone/PR naloxone in daily doses up to 80 mg/40 mg appears effective and safe [83]. Analgesia is effective while bowel function and quality of life improved with PR oxycodone/PR naloxone (20 mg/10 mg to 40 mg/20 mg) treatment in patients with severe neuropathic non–malignant pain [84]. Even at quite high doses, PR oxycodone/PR naloxone doses exhibited a benefit compared to PR oxycodone administered alone [85]. PR oxycodone/PR naloxone in doses up to 120 mg/60 mg per day provides effective analgesia while improving bowel function [76]. Adverse effects of PR oxycodone/PR naloxone and PR oxycodone are similar; the frequency of diarrhea is slightly higher in PR oxycodone/PR naloxone compared to PR oxycodone administered alone (5.2% vs. 2.6%) [81]. However, PR oxycodone/PR naloxone less frequency induces nausea (6.3% vs. 10.5%), vomiting (1.3% vs. 4.3%), abdominal pain (1.3% vs. 4.3%) and dyspepsia (0.6% vs. 2.5%) in comparison to PR oxycodone administered alone [82]. These differences might be explained by naloxone antagonist effect on gastric and gut opioid receptors and in consequence, naloxone prokinetic properties [86]. PR oxycodone/PR naloxone studies were performed mainly in patients with chronic, non–malignant pain [80–83,85,89]. Opioid switch to PR oxycodone/PR naloxone for cancer patients generally provides adequate analgesia and improved bowel function [87], but in some requiring heightened analgesia, very high doses of PR up to 240 mg per day oxycodone administered alone may be necessary[88].

The contraindications for PR oxycodone/PR naloxone comprise bowel obstruction, acute abdominal conditions, diarrhea and an allergy to the drug. PR oxycodone/PR naloxone is available in several European countries. One pack contains 60 PR oxycodone/PR naloxone tablets of 5 mg/2.5 mg, 10 mg/5 mg, 20 mg/10 mg, 40 mg/20 mg strength. Direct treatment costs for PR oxycodone/PR naloxone in patients with moderate–to–severe non–malignant pain and opioid–induced constipation is slightly higher compared to oxycodone PR. When analysing constipation treatment costs and benefits of PR oxycodone/PR naloxone in terms of improved quality–adjusted life–years, PR oxycodone/PR naloxone appears to be cost–effective option in the UK [90]. Government and other insurance schemes however may not reimburse PR oxycodone/PR naloxone tablets.

4.6. Purely peripherally acting opioid receptor antagonists

Methylnaltrexone (MNTX), a derivative of naltrexone, is a peripheral μ–opioid receptor antagonist, which does not cross blood–brain barrier [91]. Because of its low oral bioavailability, MNTX is administered subcutaneously or intravenously [92]. However, MNTX taken orally prevents the delay in oro–ceacal transit time that follows intravenous morphine administration [93]. MNTX plasma half–life equals 105 to 140 minutes. 50% is excreted unchanged in the urine. MNTX is a weak CYP2D6 inhibitor with no significant drug interactions [94]. MNTX is used to treat OIC in adult patients with advanced diseases when constipation does not respond to conventional oral laxatives. The drug is available in ampoules containing 12 mg MNTX bromide in the volume of 0.6 ml and is applied via subcutaneous injections. The recommended single MNTX dose is 8 mg in patients with body weight 38–61 kg or 12 mg if the body mass is 62–114 kg [95]. Those falling outside of this range should receive a dose of 0.15 mg/kg. No dose adjustment is necessary for patients with mild to moderate hepatic or renal impairment. However, in patients with severe renal failure (creatinine clearance < 30 mL/min) the MNTX dose should be reduced by one–half [96].

A bowel movement within 4 h after MNTX injection is observed in 50–60% patients (the median time to bowel movement after the drug administration is 30 minutes). If no therapeutic effect is observed, the injection may be repeated every other day. MNTX adverse effects comprise abdominal pain (28% of the treated patients), flatulence (13%), nausea (11%), dizziness (7%) and diarrhoea (5%) [16]. However, the administration of MNTX may be associated with an increased risk of gastrointestinal perforation in patients with diseases that decrease gut wall integrity (cancer, peptic ulceration and Ogilvie's syndrome) or on concomitant medications (NSAIDs, bevacizumab). GI perforation occur at different possible locations (duodenum, small and large bowel). A possible contributing factor might be the prokinetic effect of MNTX. It is not known if dose and duration of the treatment with MNTX relate to this complication [95]. As MNTX does not cross the blood–brain barrier, there is no attenuation of analgesia nor is there an opioid withdrawal syndrome [17]. The use of MNTX is contraindicated in patients with mechanical bowel obstruction, in acute abdominal conditions and in case of allergy to the drug. MNTX may be used in palliative care patients with OIBD not amenable to the treatment with oral laxatives. Several clinical studies have demonstrated the effectiveness of MNTX in patients with advanced diseases and with OIBD [16,17,95,96,98–100]. Peripherally active opioid receptor antagonists in the treatment of OIBD are effective and safe in [101-4]. Long–term efficacy and safety of opioid antagonists is not yet clearly established, in part due to a limited number of randomized studies [105-6].].

The Expert Working Group of the Polish Association for Palliative Medicine developed a three step ladder for the management of OIC (Fig. 1) [43]. This updated version of the ladder takes into account new therapies directed at the underlying mechanism of OIBD [107].

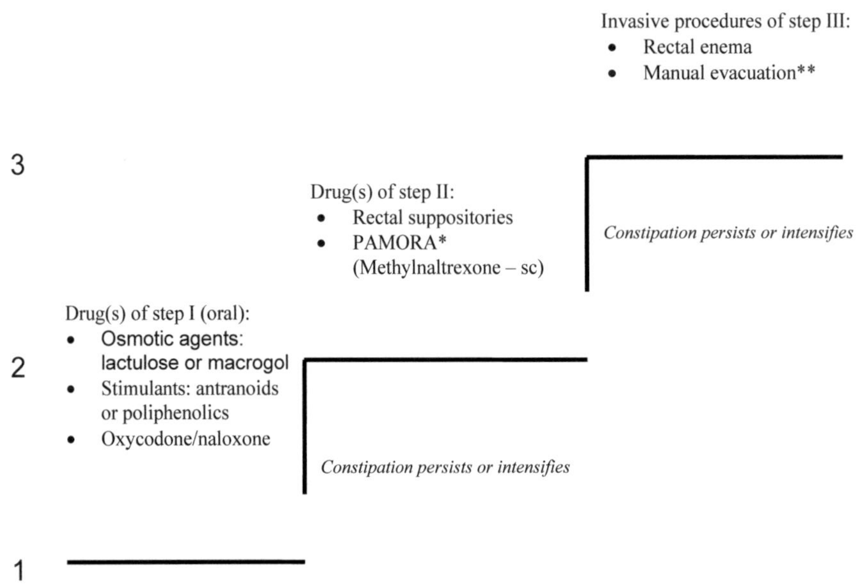

* PAMORA–peripherally acting mu–opioid receptor antagonists (methylnaltrexone) indicated for patients who do not respond to traditional oral laxatives without bowel obstruction and acute abdominal illness; ** This procedure should be used only when other measures fail and the faecal impaction causes significant pain and distress for the patient. It should be proceeded by a sedative and analgesics (local and systemic) administration that provide effective relief of severe pain and distress associated with manual stool evacuation; sc – subcutaneous

Figure 1. The three-step ladder of the management of opioid–induced constipation [43,107]

http://dx.doi.org/10.5772/56624

At the first step traditional oral laxatives and/or PR oxycodone/PR naloxone may be considered. PR oxycodone/PR naloxone targets the source of OIBD (prevention and treatment) as PR naloxone blocks opioid receptors in the gut and PR oxycodone provides effective analgesia. PR oxycodone/PR naloxone may be considered in cancer pain patients who are at high risk of OIBD development such as those with GI tumors, patients who require combined treatment with opioids and other drugs disturbing normal bowel function, e.g. advanced cancer patients. At the second step subcutaneous administration of MNTX may be considered when traditional oral laxatives are ineffective, which may allow avoiding invasive and often painful invasive procedures at step 3 of the ladder.

5. Conclusions

OIBD in patients diagnosed with chronic diseases is a challenging problem that health care providers often underestimate. This is particularly important in patients regularly receiving opioids for pain or other indications. Thanks to newly introduced drugs that target the cause of OIBD, a more effective therapy is available. The experience with MNTX and PR oxycodone/PR naloxone in patients suffering from OIBD is promising. Further clinical studies are needed to develop more effective guidelines for the management of OIBD and to establish more precisely the role of opioid receptor antagonists. The role of opioid receptor antagonists as potential antiemetic and prokinetic agents should be further explored as suggested by experimental studies in animals. The cost-benefit from new therapies must be carefully considered; overall resources may actually be saved from reduced use of traditional laxatives. The most important advantage of targeted therapies is to decrease patient suffering from OIBD, substantial reduce the need to perform invasive rectal procedures and most importantly, improve quality of life.

Author details

Wojciech Leppert*

Address all correspondence to: wojciechleppert@wp.pl

Chair and Department of Palliative Medicine, Poznan University of Medical Sciences, Poznan, Poland

References

[1] Ueberral MA, Mueller–Schwefe G. Opioid–induced constipation – a frequent and distressing side effect in daily practice affecting oral and transdermal opioid applications. Eur J Pain 2006; 10: S172.

[2] Bell TJ, Panchal SJ, Miaskowski C, Bolge SC, Milanova T, Williamson R. The Prevalence, Severity, and Impact of Opioid-Induced Bowel Dysfunction: Results of a US and European Patient Survey (PROBE 1). Pain Med 2009; 10: 35–42.

[3] Reimer K, Hopp M, Zenz M et al. Meeting the Challenges of Opioid-Induced Constipation in Chronic Pain Management – A Novel Approach. Pharmacology 2009; 83: 10–17.

[4] Davis MP. The opioid bowel syndrome: a review of pathophysiology and treatment. J Opioid Manage 2005; 1: 153–161.

[5] Holzer P. Treatment of opioid-induced gut dysfunction. Expert Opin Investig Drugs 2007; 16: 181–194.

[6] Holzer P. Opioids and opioid receptors in the myenteric nervous system: from a problem in opioid analgesia to a possible new prokinetic therapy in humans. Neurosci Lett 2004; 361: 192–195.

[7] Shook JE, Pelton JT, Hruby VJ, Burks TF. Peptide opioid antagonist separates peripheral and central opioid antitransit effects. J Pharmacol Exp Ther 1987; 243: 492–500.

[8] Sykes NP. Constipation and diarrhoea. In: Doyle D, Hanks G, Cherny N, Calman K, eds. Oxford Textbook of Palliative Medicine. Oxford University Press; Oxford 2004, pp. 483–496.

[9] Basta S, Anderson DL. Mechanisms and Management of Constipation in the Cancer Patient. J Pharmaceut Care Pain Symptom Control 1998; 6: 21–40.

[10] Potter J, Wagg A. Management of bowel problems in older people: an update. Clin Med 2005; 5: 289–295.

[11] Mumford SP. Can high fibre diets improve the bowel function in patients on radiotherapy ward? In: Twycross RG, Lack SA eds. Control of alimentary symptoms in far advanced cancer. Churchill Livingstone; Edinburgh 1986: 183.

[12] Porecca F, Cowan A, Raffa RB, Tallarida RJ. Ketazocines and morphine: effects on gastrointestinal transit after central and peripheral administration. Life Sci 1983; 32: 1785–1790.

[13] Parolado D, Sala M, Gori E. Effect of intracerebroventricular administration of morphine upon intestinal motility in rat and its antagonism with naloxone. Eur J Pharmacol 1977; 46: 329–338.

[14] Stewart JJ, Weisbrodt NW, Burks TF. Central and peripheral action of morphine on intestinal transit. J Pharmacol Exp Ther 1978; 205: 547–555.

[15] Thörn SE, Wattwil M, Lindberg G, Säwe J. Systemic and central effects of morphine on gastrointestinal motility. Acta Anaesthesiol Scand 1996; 40: 177–186.

http://dx.doi.org/10.5772/56624

[16] Thomas J, Karver S, Cooney GA et al. Methylnaltrexone for Opioid-Induced Constipation in Advanced Illness. N Engl J Med 2008; 358: 2332–2343.

[17] Slatkin N, Thomas J, Lipman AG et al. Methylnaltrexone for Treatment of Opioid–Induced Constipation in Advanced Illness Patients. J Support Oncol 2009; 7: 39–46.

[18] Wood JD, Galligan JJ. Function of opioids in the enteric nervous system. Neurogastroenterol Motil 2004; 16 (suppl. 2): 181–194.

[19] Davies MP, Walsh D. Gastrointestinal motility disorders. In: Ripamonti C, Bruera E, eds. Gastrointestinal Symptoms in Advanced Cancer Patients. Oxford University Press; Oxford 2002, pp. 127–168.

[20] Regnard C. Dysphagia, dyspepsia, and hiccup. In: Hanks G,Cherny NI, Christiakis NA, Fallon M, Kaasa S, Portenoy RK, eds. Oxford Textbook of Palliative Medicine. Oxford University Press; Oxford 2011, pp. 812–833.

[21] Narducci F, Bassotti G, Granata MT, Gaburri M, Farroni F, Palumbo R, Morelli A. Functional dyspepsia and chronic idiopathic gastric stasis. Role of endogenous opiates. Arch Intern Med 1986; 146: 716–720.

[22] Aktas A, Caner B, Ozturk F, Bayhan H, Narin Y, Mentes T. The effect of trimebutine maleate on gastric emptying in patients with non–ulcer dyspepsia. Ann Nucl Med 1999; 13: 231–234.

[23] Revicki DA, Rentz AM, Dubois D, Kahrilas P, Stanghellini V, Talley NJ, Tack J. Development and validation of a patient–assessed gastroparesis symptom severity measure: the Gastroparesis Cardinal Symptom Index. Aliment Pharm Ther 2003; 18: 141–150.

[24] Wo JM, Parkman HP. Motility and Functional Disorders of the Stomach: Diagnosis and Management of Functional Dyspepsia and Gastroparesis. Pract Gastroenterol 2006; 30: 23–48.

[25] Desta Z, Wu GM, Morocho AM, Flockhart DA. The gastroprokinetic and antiemetic drug metoclopramide is a substrate and inhibitor of cytochrome P450 2D6. Drug Metabol Dis 2002; 30: 336-343.

[26] Glare P, Nikolova T, Tickoo R, Miller J, Bras M. An overview of anti–emetic medications and the considerations for their use in palliative care. Eur J Palliat Care 2012; 19: 162–167.

[27] Twycross R, Wilcock A. Gastro–intestinal system. In: Twycross R, Wilcock A (Editors–in–Chief). Palliative Care Formulary. Fourth Edition. Palliativedrugs.com Ltd. Nottingham 2012, pp. 1–54.

[28] Potet F, Bouyssou T, Escande D, Baro I. Gastrointestinal prokinetic drugs have different affinity for the human cardiac ether–a–gogo K (+) channel. J Pharmacol Exp Ther 2001; 299: 1007–1012.

[29] Chojnacki J. Itopride in the treatment of kinetic disorders of gastrointestinal tract (in Polish). Przegl Gastroentorol 2011; 6: 139–145.

[30] Bouras EP, Camilleri M, Burton DD, Thomforde G, McKinzie S, Zinsmeister AR. Prucalopride accelerates gastrointestinal and colonic transit in patients with constipation without a rectal evacuation disorder. Gastroenterology 2001; 120: 354–360.

[31] Tack J, van Outryve M, Beyens G, Kerstens R, Vandeplassche L. Prucalopride (Resolor) in the treatment of severe chronic constipation in patients dissatisfied with laxatives. Gut 2009; 58: 357–365.

[32] Quigley EMM. Prucalopride: safety, efficacy and potential applications. Ther Adv Gastroenterol 2012; 5: 23–30.

[33] Müller–Lissner S. Pharmacokinetic and pharmacodynamic considerations for the current chronic constipation treatments. Exp Opin Drug Metabol Toxicol 2013; 9: 391–401.

[34] Bushby RW, Kessler MM, Bartolini WP. et al. Pharmacologic properties, metabolism, and disposition of linaclotide, a novel therapeutic peptide approved for the treatment of irritable bowel syndrome with constipation and chronic idiopathic constipation. J Pharmacol Exp Ther 2013; 344: 196–206.

[35] Benson AB, Stein R. Diarrhoea and Constipation: Supportive Oncology Management. In: Ettinger DS, ed. Supportive Care in Cancer Therapy. Humana Press; New York 2009, pp. 213–225.

[36] Klaschik E, Nauck F, Ostgathe C. Constipation – modern laxative therapy. Support Care Cancer 2003; 11: 679–685.

[37] Bruera E, Brenneis C, Michand M, MacDonald N. Continuous subcutaneous infusion of metoclopramide for treatment of narcotic bowel syndrome. Cancer Treat Rep 1987; 71: 1121–1122.

[38] Larkin PJ, Sykes NP, Centeno C et al. The management of constipation in palliative care: clinical practice recommendations. Palliat Med 2008; 22: 796–807.

[39] Leppert W. The management of patients with gastrointestinal symptoms in palliative care (in Polish). Terapia 2011; 19: 59–66.

[40] Mancini I, Bruera E. Constipation. In: Ripamonti C, Bruera E, eds. Gastrointestinal symptoms in advanced cancer patients. Oxford University Press; Oxford 2004: pp. 193–206.

[41] Sykes NP. Current approaches to the management of constipation. Cancer Surv 1994; 21: 137–146.

[42] Mancini I, Bruera E. Constipation in advanced cancer patients. Support Care Cancer 1998; 6: 356–364.

[43] Leppert W, Dzierzanowski T, Cialkowska–Rysz A, Jarosz J, Pyszkowska J, Stachowiak A. The management of constipation in palliative medicine – recommendations of the Expert Working Group of the Polish Association for Palliative Medicine (in Polish). Med Paliat 2009; 1: 1–10.

[44] Twycross R, Wilcock A, Toller CS. Faecal Impaction. In: Twycross R, Wilcock A, Toller CS. Symptom Management in Advanced Cancer. Palliativedrugs.com Ltd, Nottingham 2009, pp. 119–120.

[45] Wirz S, Nadstawek J, Elsen C, Junker U, Wartenberg HC. Laxative management in ambulatory cancer patients on opioid therapy: a prospective, open–label investigation of polyethylene glycol, sodium picosulphate and lactulose. Eur J Cancer Care 2012: 21: 131–140.

[46] Belsey D, Geraint M, Dixon TA. Systematic review and meta analysis: polyethylene glycol in adults with non–organic constipation. Int J Clin Pract 2010; 64: 944–955.

[47] Miles CL, Fellowes D, Goodman ML, Wilkinson S. Laxatives for the management of constipation in palliative care patients. Cochrane Database Syst Rev 2011; (1): CD003448.

[48] Mercadante S, Bruera E. Opioid switching: a systematic and critical review. Cancer Treat Rev 2006; 32: 304–315.

[49] Leppert W. Progress in pharmacological pain treatment with opioid analgesics (in Polish). Wspolcz Onkol 2009; 13: 66–73.

[50] Ahmedzai S, Brooks D. Transdermal Fentanyl versus Sustained–Release Oral Morphine in Cancer Pain: Preference, Efficacy and Quality of Life. J Pain Symptom Manage 1997; 13: 254–261.

[51] Haazen L, Noorduin H, Megens A, Meert T. The constipation–inducing potential of morphine and transdermal fentanyl. Eur J Pain 1999; 3 (Suppl. A): 9–15.

[52] Hunt R, Fazekas B, Thorne D, Brooksbank M. A comparison of subcutaneous morphine and fentanyl in hospice cancer patients. J Pain Symptom Manage 1999; 18: 111–119.

[53] Tassinari D, Sartori S, Tamburini E et al. Adverse Effects of Transdermal Opiates Treating Moderate–Severe Cancer Pain in Comparison to Long–Acting Morphine: A Meta–Analysis and Systematic Review of the Literature. J Palliat Med 2008; 11: 492–502.

[54] Rosti G, Gatti A, Costantini A, Sabato AF, Zucco F. Opioid–related bowel dysfunction: prevalence and identification of predictive factors in a large sample of Italian patients on chronic treatment. Eur Rev Med Pharmacol Sci 2010; 14: 1045–1050.

[55] Weschules DJ, Bain KT, Reifsnyder J, et al. Toward Evidence–Based Prescribing at End of Life: A Comparative Analysis of Sustained–Release Morphine, Oxycodone,

and Transdermal Fentanyl, with Pain, Constipation, and Caregiver Interaction Outcomes in Hospice Patients. Pain Med 2006; 7: 320–329.

[56] Bach V, Kamp–Jensen M, Jensen N–H, Eriksen J. Buprenorphine and sustained release oral morphine – effect and side–effects in chronic use. Pain Clin 1991; 4: 87–93.

[57] Mancini IL, Hanson J, Neumann CM, Bruera E. Opioid type and other clinical predictors of laxative dose in advanced cancer patients: a retrospective study. J Palliat Med 2000; 3: 49–56.

[58] Daeninck PJ, Bruera E. Reduction in constipation and laxative requirements following opioid rotation to methadone: a report of four cases. J Pain Symptom Manage 1999; 18: 303–309.

[59] Mercadante S, Casuccio A, Fulfaro F et al. Switching From Morphine to Methadone to Improve Analgesia and Tolerability in Cancer Patients: A Prospective Study. J Clin Oncol 2001; 19: 2898–2904.

[60] Grond S, Radbruch L, Meuser T, Loick G, Sabatowski R, Lehmann KA. High–Dose Tramadol in Comparison to Low–Dose Morphine for Cancer Pain Relief. J Pain Symptom Manage 1999; 18: 174–179.

[61] Duggan AK. The cost of constipation in morphine patients and the economic possibilities with tramadol. Br J Med Econom 1995; 9: 21–29.

[62] Leppert W. Analgesic efficacy and side effects of oral tramadol and morphine administered orally in the treatment of cancer pain. Nowotwory 2001; 51: 257–266.

[63] Leppert W, Majkowicz M. Assessment of analgesia and adverse effects of controlled release tramadol and dihydrocodeine in patients with cancer pain – based on a modified ESAS. Wspolcz Onkol 2008; 12: 246–254.

[64] Wirz S, Witmmann M, Schenk M et al. Gastrointestinal symptoms under opioid therapy: A prospective comparison of oral sustained–release hydromorphone, transdermal fentanyl, and transdermal buprenorphine. Eur J Pain 2009; 13: 737–743.

[65] Sykes NP. A clinical comparison of laxatives in a hospice. Palliat Med 1991; 5: 307–314.

[66] Miles CL, Fellowes D, Goodman ML, Wilkinson S. Laxatives for the management of constipation in palliative care patients. Cochrane Database Syst Rev 2006; 4: CD003448.

[67] Holzer P, Ahmedzai SH, Niederle N et al. Opioid–induced bowel dysfunction in cancer–related pain: causes, consequences, and a novel approach for its management. J Opioid Manage 2009; 5: 145–195.

[68] Sykes NP. An investigation of the ability of oral naloxone to correct opioid–related constipation in patients with advanced cancer. Palliat Med 1996; 10: 135–144.

[69] Liu M, Wittbrodt E. Low-dose oral naloxone reverses opioid–induced constipation and analgesia. J Pain Symptom Manage 2002; 23: 48–53.

[70] Meissner W, Schimdt U, Hartmann M et al. Oral naloxone reverses opioid–induced constipation. Pain 2000; 84: 105–109.

[71] Glass PS, Jhaveri RM, Smith LR. Comparison of potency and duration of action of nalmefene and naloxone. Anesth Analg 1994; 78: 536–541.

[72] Cheskin LJ, Chami TN, Johnson RE et al. Assessment of nalmefene glucuronide as a selective gut opioid antagonist. Drug Alcohol Depend 1995; 39: 151–154.

[73] Nadstawek J, Leyendecker P, Hopp M et al. Patient assessment of a novel therapeutic approach for the treatment of severe, chronic pain. Int J Clin Pract 2008; 62: 1159–1167.

[74] Leyendecker P, Hopp M, Bosse B et al. Bowel Function Index (BFI), a new validated questionnaire for assessing opioid induced constipation. Proceedings of the IASP Congress on Pain, Glasgow; 2008.

[75] Anonim. Oxycodone/naloxone prolonged release tablets, questions and answers. Paineurope supplement. February 2009.

[76] Ahmedzai SH, Nauck F, Bar–Sela G, Bosse B, Leyendecker P, Hopp M. A randomized, double–blind, active–controlled, double–dummy, parallel–group study to determine the safety and efficacy of oxycodone/naloxone prolonged-release tablets in patients with moderate/severe, chronic cancer pain. Palliat Med 2012; 26: 50–60.

[77] Kalso E. Oxycodone. J Pain Symptom Manage 2005; 29 (5S): S47–S56.

[78] Biancofiore G. Oxycodone controlled release in cancer pain management. Therap Clinic Risk Manage 2006; 2: 228–234.

[79] Fishman J, Roffwarg H, Helman L. Disposition of naloxone–7,8–3H in normal and narcotic–dependent men. J Pharmacol Exp Ther 1973; 187: 575–580.

[80] Müller–Lissner S, Leyendecker P, Hopp M, Ruckes C, Fleischer W, Reimer K. Oral prolonged release (PR) oxycodone/naloxone combination reduces opioid–induced bowel dysfunction (OIBD) in patients with severe chronic pain. Eur J Pain 2007; 11 (S82): abstract 189.

[81] Vondrackova D, Leyendecker P, Meissner W et al. Analgesic Efficacy and Safety of Oxycodone in Combination With Naloxone as Prolonged Release Tablets in Patients With Moderate to Severe Chronic Pain. J Pain 2008; 9: 1144–1154.

[82] Simpson K, Leyendecker P, Hopp M et al. Fixed–ratio combination oxycodone/naloxone compared with oxycodone alone for the relief of opioid–induced constipation in moderate–to–severe noncancer pain. Curr Med Res Opin 2008; 24: 3503–3512.

[83] Sandner–Kiesling A, Leyendecker P, Hopp M et al. Long–term efficacy and safety of combined prolonged-release oxycodone and naloxone in the management of non-cancer chronic pain. Int J Clin Pract 2010; 64: 763–774.

[84] Hermanns K, Junker U, Nolte T. Prolonged–release oxycodone/naloxone in the treatment of neuropathic pain – results from a large observational study. Exp Opin Pharmacother 2012; 13: 299–311.

[85] Löwenstein O, Leyendecker P, Hopp M et al. Combined prolonged release oxycodone and naloxone improves bowel function in patients receiving opioids for moderate–to–severe non–malignant chronic pain: a randomized controlled trial. Expert Opin Pharmacother 2009; 10: 531–453.

[86] Schang JC, Devroede G. Beneficial effects of naloxone in a patient with intestinal pseudoobstruction. Am J Gastroenterol 1985; 80: 407–411.

[87] Clemens KE, Quednau I, Klaschik E. Bowel function during pain therapy with oxycodone/naloxone prolonged-release tablets in patients with advanced cancer. Int J Clin Pract 2011; 65: 472–478.

[88] Mercadante S, Ferrera P, Adile C. High doses of oxycodone–naloxone combination may provide poor analgesia. Support Care Cancer 2011; 19: 1471–1472.

[89] Meissner W, Leyendecker P, Meuller–Lissner S et al. A randomised controlled trial with prolonged–release oral oxycodone and naloxone to prevent and reverse opioid–induced constipation. Eur J Pain 2009; 13: 56–64.

[90] Dunlop W, Uhl R, Khan I, Taylor A, Barton G. Quality of life benefits and cost impact of prolonged release oxycodone/naloxone versus prolonged release oxycodone in patients with moderate–to–severe non–malignant pain and opioid–induced constipation: a UK cost–utility analysis. J Med Econ 2012; 15: 564–575.

[91] Shaiova L, Rim F, Friedman D, Jahdi M. A review of methylnaltrexone, a peripheral opioid receptor antagonist, and its role in opioid–induced constipation. Palliat Support Care 2007; 5: 161–166.

[92] Yuan CS. Clinical Status of Methylnaltrexone, A New Agent to Prevent and Manage Opioid–Induced Side Effects. J Support Oncol 2004; 2: 111–122.

[93] Yuan CS, Foss JF, Osinski J, Toledano A, Roizen MF, Moss J. The safety and efficacy of oral Clinical methylnaltrexone in preventing morphine–induced delay in oral–cecal transit time. Clin Pharmacol Ther 1997; 61: 467–475.

[94] Abarca FM, Saclarides TJ, Brand MI. A Review of the Treatment of Opioid–induced Constipation with Methylnaltrexone Bromide. Clinical Medicine Insights: Therapeutics 2010; 2: 53–60.

[95] Portenoy RK, Thomas J, Moehl Boathwright ML. et al. Subcutaneous methylnaltrexone for the treatment of opioid-induced constipation in patients with advanced ill-

ness: a double–blind, randomized, parallel group, dose–ranging study. J Pain Symptom Manage 2008; 35: 458–468.

[96] Chamberlain BH, Cross K, Winston JL et al. Methylnaltrexone Treatment of Opioid–Induced Constipation in Patients with Advanced Illness. J Pain Symptom Manage 2009; 38: 683–690.

[97] Corken A, Green L, Greene P, Avigan M. Methylnatrexone and Gastrointestinal Perforation. J Pain Symptom Manage 2010; 40: e1–e3.

[98] Becker G, Galandi D, Blum HE. Peripherally Acting Opioid Antagonists in the Treatment of Opiate–Related Constipation: a Systematic Review. J Pain Symptom Manage 2007; 34: 547–565.

[99] Yuan CS. Methylnaltrexone mechanisms of action and side effects on opioid bowel dysfunction and of the opioid adverse effects. Ann Pharmacother 2007; 41: 984–993.

[100] Yuan CS, Foss JF, O'Connor M et al. Methylnaltrexone for Reversal of Constipation Due to Chronic Methadone Use: A Randomized Controlled Trial. JAMA 2000; 283: 367–372.

[101] McNicol E, Boyce DB, Schumann R, Carr D. Efficacy and Safety of Mu–Opioid Antagonists in the Treatment of Opioid–Induced Bowel Dysfunction: Systematic Review and Meta–analysis of Randomized Controlled Trials. Pain Med 2008; 9: 634–659.

[102] McNicol ED, Boyce D, Schumann R, Carr DB. Mu-opioid antagonists for opioid–induced bowel dysfunction. Cochrane Database Syst Rev. 2008 Apr 16; (2):CD006332.

[103] Paulson DM, Kennedy DT, Donovick RA et al. Alvimopan: An oral, peripherally acting, mu–opioid receptor antagonist for the treatment of opioid–induced bowel dysfunction – a 21–day treatment–randomized trial. J Pain 2005; 6: 184–192.

[104] Leppert W. The role of opioid receptor antagonists in the treatment of opioid-induced constipation – a review. Adv Ther 2010; 27: 714–730.

[105] Leppert W. The impact of opioid analgesics on the gastrointestinal tract function and the current management possibilities. Wspolcz Onkol 2012; 16: 125–131.

[106] Candy B, Jones L, Goodman ML, Drake R, Tookman A. Laxatives or methylnaltrexone for the management of constipation in palliative care patients. Cochrane Database Syst Rev 2011; 1: CD003448.

[107] Leppert W. The place of oxycodone/naloxone in chronic pain management. Wspolcz Onkol 2013; 17: 128–133